EBURY P

HEALED

Manisha Koirala is one of India's leading film actors. Born into the prominent Koirala family of Nepal, she made her Bollywood debut with *Saudagar* in 1991, before going on to establish herself as one of the leading actresses with films such as *1942: A Love Story*, *Akele Hum Akele Tum*, *Bombay*, *Khamoshi: The Musical*, *Dil Se*, *Mann*, *Lajja* and *Company*. She took a break from acting in 2012 and returned five years later with the coming-of-age drama *Dear Maya*, Netflix's *Lust Stories* and *Sanju*. She was appointed the Goodwill Ambassador for the United Nations Population Fund in 1999 and 2015, and was involved in the relief work following the Nepal earthquake in 2015. She promotes causes such as women's rights, prevention of violence against women, prevention of human trafficking and cancer awareness. She was diagnosed with ovarian cancer in 2012 and has been cancer-free since 2013.

Neelam Kumar is a bestselling author, motivational speaker, soft-skills trainer and life-skills coach. This is her ninth book. She lives in Mumbai and can be reached at corporate.lounge@gmail.com as well as through her website, www.neelamkumar.in.

PRAISE FOR *HEALED*

'*Healed* has both the raw truth of a journal, the sort you write when you know no one's reading; and the wisdom of experience, the kind you put out when you know people are listening, and that they will hear your voice'—*The Hindu*

'*Healed* is a deeply personal account of the actor's struggle with cancer and her triumph over it. It is also a heartbreaking portrait of a once-upon-a-time superstar, narrated with disarming honesty'—*Indian Express*

'Books on disease and disability haven't produced many best-sellers in India. Now, with more openness about issues of the body and survivor stories, with an emphasis on positivity, which an ever-growing wellness industry endorses, a book like *Healed* is a best-seller idea. We live in a world that thrives on the promise of self-improvement, cleansing and healing, and memoirs of someone who has overcome the biggest of all maladies and healed from its after-effects is an abiding story. We see a sensitive, vulnerable and deeply empathetic person entrenched in the faith of companionship and human bonding in these chapters, and it is a triumph of self-expression'—Livemint

'It is a book of self-discovery, where the author honestly and minutely analyses her own life, her decisions, her "toxic relationships" and mistakes. It combs through events and people that shaped her, and allowed her to overcome the disease. The fluid narrative borrows on memories of an actress who has starred in over 80 Bollywood movies, and lays bare the ordinary human being behind the trappings of the spotlight and glamour. Nothing is spared, the raw emotions are laid out in agonising detail: her post surgery "ruthlessly stapled" abdomen, the time she lets out a "guttural cry" in the privacy of her shower, or when she likens the agony of the first chemotherapy session to ". . . dark, wild wolves, their mouths open, fangs bared, seeking out each vein of my body, tearing forward at great speed, hell-bent on destruction"'—*Nepali Times*

HEALED

How cancer gave me a new life

MANISHA KOIRALA

with NEELAM KUMAR

EBURY
PRESS

An imprint of Penguin Random House

EBURY PRESS

USA | Canada | UK | Ireland | Australia
New Zealand | India | South Africa | China

Ebury Press is part of the Penguin Random House group of companies
whose addresses can be found at global.penguinrandomhouse.com

Published by Penguin Random House India Pvt. Ltd
4th Floor, Capital Tower 1, MG Road,
Gurugram 122 002, Haryana, India

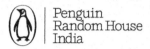

First published in Viking by Penguin Random House India 2018
Published in Ebury Press 2022

10 9 8 7 6 5 4 3 2 1

The views and opinions expressed in this book are the author's own and the
facts are as reported by her which have been verified to the extent possible,
and the publishers are not in any way liable for the same.

ISBN 9780143457206

Typeset in RequiemText by Manipal Digital Systems, Manipal

www.penguin.co.in

To you, dear reader.

May you realize your limitless human potential and rekindle your inner spirit to face every challenge life throws at you.

Contents

Preface   ix

Prologue   xi

1. That Sinking Feeling   1
2. Kathmandu   5
3. Mumbai   17
4. New York   37
5. Meeting Dr Chi   47
6. Broken, but Picked Up by Love   51
7. Surgery   61
8. Dr Makker Enters My Life   71
9. How Bollywood Came to My Rescue   77
10. New Apartment Joys   89
11. Chemotherapy   95
12. Cancer-Free   117
13. Stepping Out—Fearfully   123
14. Team Mumbai   129
15. Home to Kathmandu and Chaos Again   143

16. Vulnerability—The Chink in My Armour   153

17. Birthing the New Me in My Sanctuary   159

18. Lessons Learnt, Wisdom Passed On   173

19. Cancer as My Gift   183

20. Not Only through the Male Gaze   195

21. Living the New Me   205

Epilogue   211

Acknowledgements   213

Books and Resources: My Portable Magic   217

Preface

In 2013, while I was battling cancer in New York, I met a Rinpoche who had travelled to the US from Nepal. In Tibetan, Rinpoche means the 'precious one'. It is an honorific title used in Tibetan Buddhism for a teacher of the dharma.

He advised me to treat every feeling I was going through as a 'precious jewel' and pen all of them down while I was experiencing them. He further told me that the mind was conditioned to forget and if I did not commit these feelings and thoughts to paper, I would lose the valuable lessons of my chemotherapy days in the mundaneness of everyday life.

So while going through that phase of my life I kept fragmented notes in my diary, hoping to spin them into a book later. Truth be told, bits of this book were written in my head during my chemo days. But I found it hard to sit down with my painful memories and document them in a book.

Now I have finally got around to writing one. My book is a result of intense soul-searching. I have plunged deep into the dark, bottomless pit of painful memories and woven a story out of them. It has taken a lot of courage to confront and relive my experiences. But I needed to do so in order to become a true storyteller for the readers' sake as well as my own.

Manisha means Saraswati. This book is an attempt to look for the Saraswati in Manisha.

Writing it has been a soulful experience for me. And I hope it will make an enjoyable read for you.

I offer my book to you with a lot of love.

Prologue

'I don't want to die,' I texted my friend in desperation.

The feeling of being engulfed by darkness was fast descending on me. Even as I choked and struggled to fight it, darkness clutched at my throat, cutting off the light. Then it travelled swiftly, sweeping ruthlessly through my body, and finally settled into the pit of my stomach.

I panicked at the old memory of feeling abandoned.

It had happened to me at age eight when my mother left me at my grandmother's house in Benares and simply walked away. Wide-eyed, I had remained standing there, waiting for her to look back and take me in her arms. She never did.

'Why didn't you turn?' I asked her many years later.

'Because, my little one, I did not want you to see me get teary-eyed.'

It was only years later that I understood why she had left me there. She was helping out my father in Nepal's mounting political activities and knew that my grandmother, who had ably raised several children, would look after me well.

Of course, with time I had understood my beloved mother's situation and the wisdom of what she had done back then. But could I shake off the feeling of abandonment imprinted on my young soul? No.

I felt a similar tinge of desertion when my marriage failed. I had tried my best to make it work and its collapse weighed heavily on my soul. But we were just two very different people— not meant to be with each other. Why did I always end up choosing the wrong guy? I fretted over what the world would say. That I could not even handle a marriage well?

The fear of being abandoned had chased me all my life.

This fear, however, was unlike anything I had experienced before.

It was the fear of being abandoned by life itself.

I

That Sinking Feeling

'Uncertainty is life's way of saying that there are only a few things you can control.'

—Anonymous

10 December 2012

It was a cold winter morning at the Memorial Sloan Kettering Cancer Center in New York.

I remember how the frost settled on the windowpanes, blocking my view of what I imagined must be a winter wonderland. Snowflakes fell gently on the barren trees, covering them protectively like a soft eiderdown, and lulled them to sleep until they were ready to bloom again. Christmas was just around the corner.

I imagined children laughing and running in the squishy undergrowth, families decorating their Christmas trees with fairy lights, lovers snuggling up to each other with renewed promises. It was the season of love and newness.

The stark contrast of my situation hit me like a blow. I was alone in my room at the hospital, feeling empty and broken. From the high life of a Bollywood star, I had suddenly been reduced to a patient battling for life.

Death was staring me in the face. Was I going to be just another statistic?

I don't want to die, I sobbed out to the pristine white ceiling. But it just stared back at me.

Yet again my heart became a fierce battleground for life and death. Optimism and despair. The endless tug-of-war kept playing out in my mind.

You, Manisha, are going to live through this, Hope reassured me.

But you are BRCA-1 positive and have stage-III ovarian cancer, Death hissed back.

There is a 44 per cent survival rate in such cases, Hope soothed me.

There is a 56 per cent chance of you dying, Death jeered back.

I shut my eyes to let the voices fade away. It was comforting to sink into nothingness.

Whenever I needed comfort, my heart would fly to the visually stunning images of my country, Nepal. I found myself wanting to soak in the majesty of the snow-covered peaks of the Himalayas. I remembered the moments of perfect bliss on watching the orange-and-pink glow of the fading sun splashing them with colour, before they were transformed into torches of fire. And then the sadness of the fading embers.

I found myself ambling into Kathmandu's quaint lanes, my nose assailed by the strong concoction of pungent, musty, fetid and cloyingly sweet smells of hashish, fish, vegetables and spices. The exotic smell of *jimbu*, the high-altitude herb that dominates the famous Asan market, teased my senses. I elbowed my way through the narrow streets lined with palaces, temples, shrines, stupas and pagodas—structures that stand testimony to Nepal's rich heritage of art, culture and its ancient history.

My eyes felt dazzled by the riot of reds, oranges, pale-goldens and deep-browns. The fragrance of the magnolia flower teased my senses. I felt wrapped in the memory of a favourite childhood smell—that of lavender and honey. My eyes swept through Nepal's endless lush greenery that I enjoyed during my Shivpuri and other treks on the outskirts of Kathmandu Valley. Despite the ugliness of modern construction, Nepal still remained a veritable Mother's Store for me—soothing, relaxing and pure.

I have always felt that if you cut me up, you will find in my veins the roar of the mighty Bagmati of Nepal and the majestic Ganges of India—for my life has played out in these two beautiful countries. Though born into the politically prominent Koirala family, several of whose members have gone on to rule the nation, I made India my land of choice. I lived the stuff of dreams in magical Mumbai, acting in eighty-plus films, emerging as a top Bollywood heroine of my times and winning many coveted awards over the years.

I am deeply grateful for all that but the journey has been far from smooth. The canvas of my heart has registered each emotion—the delirious happiness of success . . . the despair of failed relationships . . . the shock of unexpected betrayals . . . the disbelief at the steady drying up of opportunities . . . the feeling of hopelessness upon being confronted with my diagnosis.

I did not know how much time had passed, but when I woke up, my mouth was dry. I sensed that I was in a different room. It appeared to be neither the operation nor the recovery room. My heart missed a beat. I was in a hospital room. Had I made it?

I looked up wearily and saw my mother walk in.

She is going to tell me the good news. But why is she not smiling? Why is she not meeting my eyes with that happy, tender look she always gives me?

Where is Dr Dennis Chi—my saviour? What is happening?

And then I saw him walk in.

Since my diagnosis, I had perfected the art of deciphering the truth from people's faces. It frustrated me that others would often withhold crucial information from me, as a show of kindness. But I could always ferret out the truth, as body language rarely lies.

This time too, I focused hard on reading his face. I wanted the truth.

I tried reading his eyes. *Nothing.*

I tried reading his expression. *Nothing.*

That's when the truth hit me. Like a six-foot boxer's steel punch landing right in the hollow of my stomach.

My verdict had been pronounced.

Cancer had won.

I was dying.

2

Kathmandu

'I am packed with broken glass and memories and it all hurts.'
—*Henry Rollins*

November 2012

It was midnight. I was lying alone on a white hospital bed at Norvic International Hospital, Kathmandu. In the dimly lit room my mind played havoc with me. I felt cold, lonely and frightened.

I fought hard between two instincts—that of running away and of stopping myself from screaming.

The room was sparse and smelt of hospital disinfectant.

On the wall opposite me was a clock with its minute hand stuck at six.

Why am I here? Why am I not in the maternity hospital opposite the road? Why am I not admitted for pregnancy instead? Will I ever be able to hold my baby in my arms?

It's funny that when the mind is too tired of its own thoughts, the eye starts noticing mundane things.

In the sliver of moonlight sneaking in from the window, I noticed how well kept and organized my room was. While coming in, I had noticed how impressive this section of the hospital was. I wondered if this area was meant only for VIPs.

As for me, I felt exposed. Like a huge wound whose covering had just been scratched off.

For the hundredth time, I stroked my protruding stomach and silently grieved.

The circumstances leading to my visiting this hospital had had a long build-up.

While in Mumbai, I had felt constantly sick for months. I was bloated all the time. It devastated me to hear people tell me that yesteryear's slim, beautiful girl had gained weight. And it was true. I just could not stop the kilos from piling up, especially around my stomach.

I then decided to exercise vigorously. I worked out every day to get rid of what I thought back then was 'belly fat'. I began doing Pilates. I began sweating it out in the gym. The results showed and I began to lose weight from everywhere . . . except my stomach. That part of my anatomy seemed to have a mind of its own. It was on a solo trip of expansion. And I was very unhappy with the shape my body was taking.

In frustration, I visited many doctors in Mumbai, but before a thorough check-up could be done, I had to leave for Kathmandu. Actors, especially the young and desirable ones, have a horror of getting old. But now I had to admit to myself that perhaps old age was finally catching up on me. I was forty.

Three months ago, in Mumbai, I had visited the Siddhivinayak temple. I had uttered a simple prayer, quite humorous in hindsight:

Lord, please show me my path—my purpose in life. I've been piling on the kilos and nothing seems to work. Please help me get rid of this bloating.

I took a *mannat*, a vow, there that I would not touch grains, non-vegetarian food or alcohol for three months. I had heard that sadhus fasted in this manner. I was ready to try anything at this point.

In November 2012, I flew down to Kathmandu. I remember that day being a memorable one. My friend's sister was getting married. It was the perfect occasion to end my self-imposed abstinence. In hindsight, it also turned out to be just two days before my diagnosis.

Unaware of what lay ahead, I was in a celebratory mood. All my friends were drinking and enjoying themselves. I too reached for happiness—a glass of wine. To my horror, my stomach bloated up again. I was disappointed to see that my self-denial and restraint had yielded no result.

In my car, on my way to my Kathmandu home, I suddenly felt a sharp pain in the abdomen. It got worse with each bump my car took.

That entire night I lay flat on my back. I couldn't even turn on my sides. What was happening to me? I felt angry, confused and frightened.

The next morning I spoke to my brother, Siddharth, whom I lovingly call Bhai. My voice was quivering and my face was distorted with pain.

'I can't take it any more! I need this to be diagnosed.'

Acting promptly, my brother brought me to this hospital.

So here I was, waiting for the doctor and reliving my life in my head.

***

That morning, when Dr Madhu Ghimire examined me, I felt relieved. He had a distinguished air about him. His white coat had a black-rimmed pocket on the right with the hospital's initials embroidered on it. Somehow, his attire matched his salt-and-pepper hair. It felt right.

He's now going to examine me and tell me it will all be fine, I thought.

'Just an infection, Manisha. We'll handle it.'

I will finally be free of this pain and go on to enjoy the long treks in the flower-and-tree-lined pathways of Kathmandu again.

Casually, I heard myself suggest to him that it could be a liver issue as I had been drinking a bottle of wine almost every day for several months before my three-month-long fast. Ignoring my expert diagnosis, the doctor began examining my stomach.

'There is a lot of fluid in your stomach which needs to be tested.' He took a syringe and, even as I flinched, jabbed it in my abdomen and pulled it out expertly, informing me that he would send the sample for biopsy.

I was asked to remain in the hospital overnight as my CT scan was scheduled for the next morning. I became impatient. Patience has never been my greatest virtue. The next day, I was actually quite relieved when I was wheeled out for a CT scan. Imaging over, I was brought back to my hospital room.

And then began the interminable wait. Once again my imagination began working overtime.

What if they discover it is cirrhosis of the liver? What if it is something more terrible? Are you listening, Universe? Just make me well!

For the hundredth time, I asked the nurse, 'Where is Dr Ghimire? When will he come?'

And for the hundredth time she said, 'He is busy. He will come as soon as he can.'

Morning stretched into afternoon and the sun's rays dipped. Soon it was dusk. I have always found this time of the day the most dramatic of all. It is as if the stage is being set for something ominous. My patience was snapping.

Why is nobody coming with any news? Have they not sent my sample for biopsy then?

Evening was about to stretch its fingers and smother the daylight's neck. Just then my family walked in—one by one—my parents, my brother, my aunt and uncle, my cousins.

But why? Why have they all come to see me? This is very strange!

A part of me panicked. And then I spoke in a voice that was muffled by distress.

'What is it? Will someone tell me?'

My perplexed gaze fell on the doctor, who was standing right behind my family members. He came towards me with measured steps, slowly . . . oh, so slowly . . . one foot at a time. Under the glare of the solitary tube light, I could see that his salt-and-pepper hair was a little dishevelled. Did I imagine the shimmer of unshed tears in his eyes? Or were they simply tired?

His specs hung on a black string from his neck. In his hands, he held some loose papers and a file which seemed to have been turned over several times. I could see him begin to form words.

Please tell me!

'Manisha, there are treatments for these things nowadays.'

'Treatment? What do you mean by treatment?' I yelped. I was agitated, pulling at my brown neck scarf impatiently. It suddenly felt as if it were constricting me.

'It's not like earlier. Science has advanced a lot. There are various effective treatments. People do live longer.'

'But what do I have? What treatment are we discussing?'

Dr Ghimire paused briefly, as if to gather himself.

'Manisha, my dear, you have cancer!'

'C-A-N-C-E-R?' I repeated the word incredulously. 'How can I have cancer?'

I remember the sheer shock of hearing that word making me laugh with disbelief. I looked the other way. As if I were throwing away a heavy quilt. As if by shrugging it away I was disowning it. It didn't belong to me.

Others have got cancer. How could I have it? I was healthy, ate well, exercised well. No, no, there must be a mistake!

And then, gently, the doctor went on to say, 'It's late-stage ovarian cancer.'

I refused to comprehend his words. 'Why can't you just cut it off and throw it away?' After all, I had seen this happen in many films.

My aunt, a renowned gynaecologist, had earlier surprised me by looking at my stomach and asking me if I was pregnant. I had told her that it was just not possible.

Now, in her characteristically straightforward way of speaking, she said in a small, defeated voice, 'How much can we cut off? And what all? It has spread everywhere.'

From a distance, disjointed words floated towards me. Dr Ghimire was suggesting the next course of action. He said that I should be taken to the best medical centre for cancer, which he believed was in the US. But I was in a state in which my mind refused to comprehend anything.

I'm not sure I heard anything after that. The room was spinning. The ground had slipped from under me. I was at once floating and sinking. It was a strange space to be in.

From the periphery of my vision, I could see that my beloved parents had become numb with shock. My father, who is generally reticent and calm, also looked badly shaken. They stepped out of the room together, their shoulders sagging. In the corridor, they began talking in hushed whispers. I knew that I was the topic of their discussion.

I have no idea how the hours after that were spent. I kept staring at the wall. But one by one, my family members came up to me. Silence lay between us like an impenetrable bridge. Gently, they placed their arms on me and then faded into the background. No words were spoken—just a compassionate touch to let me know they were there. It was the longest and loneliest night I have ever spent.

Next morning, I could sense a different Manisha get into the family car—dishevelled, shaken and wearing the previous day's clothes. My navy-blue track pant and white T-shirt looked badly crumpled. Un-star like. But I was beyond caring.

Quickly, I put on my sunglasses to protect myself from the harsh glare of the morning sun, but more so from reality. Silence hung heavy in our car. Nobody spoke.

For one crazy moment, I longed to see the majestic peaks of the Himalayas. The car sped on. All I could see were crowded roads and the dust on them.

My eyes inadvertently fell on a fallen eucalyptus tree. It had been snapped by some onslaught, but that is not what caught my attention. The tree lay prostrate, but the branch attached to it still had bright young leaves sprouting out of it with determination.

My feelings got tangled in the electric poles with their swinging cables above, until they were lost in mid-thought. A stray hope floated into my mind: *Is it possible for life to defeat death?*

Soon, we drove into the dip in the pathway that took us into the stone-lined approach road to the wooden gate of my bungalow. I had overheard the family's plans—first at the hospital, then at my family home. They were planning to fly me to Mumbai for a second opinion. At this point I had no say in the matter. No protests to make. I was just an automaton, going with the flow. I felt sorry for myself.

All I wanted was to walk to my special place in my home—the sun-spattered wooden veranda which had hosted me during my innumerable spells of daydreaming and reading. On those occasions, I had dreamt about everything life was capable of giving me. Everything I wanted. It had been my launch pad to make plans for my wondrous life ahead. Overnight, things had changed. I was no longer in a position to make plans. I had no life to live. I felt spent.

Yet I gazed at nature's abundance around me. At this hour of the morning, the sun deck lived up to its name. In spite of myself, I began to admire the magic my mom had created there.

The garden was alive. My listless eyes took in the orange-flowered *gulmohar* trees, the vivid purplish red of the fuchsias and the pink, purple, orange, yellow, white and magenta of the bougainvillea. It was a riot of colours.

Amidst this heaven, birds of all variety chirped—brown-feathered nightingales with their red-sided tails and sprightly buff-brown sparrows with white cheeks.

As I inhaled the mesmerizing fragrance of the white jasmines, I silently saluted Mom for all the life forms she had nurtured. Not only me and my brother, but even these cherry blossoms, pine, neem, avocado, mango, banana and bamboo trees. She had reared them lovingly from young saplings to gigantic trees. I revelled in this semi-jungle. Despite my mood, I felt revived and nourished.

My family knew that in times of distress, I preferred to be left alone. And whenever I was immersed in myself, this hardwood patio was my retreat. I could stay there for hours.

My spell was broken as I sensed somebody coming up to me. It was my sister-in-law, Yulia. I looked up at her dramatically tall, slender figure. She shook her blonde hair and silently settled down beside me on the rosewood deck.

She said nothing. Just looked at my topknot and my hands that lay limp beside me. In my eyes, she could read the pain, the shock, the confusion. She could see I was grieving.

Wordlessly, she poured hot water into the two white cups containing green tea leaves and handed one over to me.

I have always admired Yulia, a Russian brought up in Kazakhstan, for the ease with which she uprooted herself from her successful corporate career in London to settle in Nepal with my brother after marriage.

Would being uprooted from my world also be as easy, I wondered.

We sipped our tea in silence until I felt obligated to speak.

'If this is the end of my life, I must accept it, Yulia.' I whispered.

'No,' said Yulia, shaking her head in strong disagreement. 'You have to try. You just have to try to give yourself a chance.'

I looked at her with eyes full of pathos.

'You must *want* to live with passion. If you are going to be defeated, you cannot come out of this like a winner.'

I looked at her in bewilderment.

Where had she hidden so much of inner strength earlier? Why did I not notice it before? Perhaps she is right. Have I really given up before even trying?

A newfound admiration for this strong woman rose within me. With a few simple words, she had nudged the deepest part of my being. She had prodded me to walk ahead instead of making a retreat.

Is it possible for me to do so? Did I have it in me?

I do not know how long I remained in that safe space, toying with every emotion that crossed my mind. But my reverie was broken when the sharp sound of a conch shell reached my ears. It came from within my home. My mother must have begun the prayer rituals.

I learnt later that my cousins had rushed to an astrologer on hearing the doctor's verdict and consulted him about my Vedic astrological chart. To their amazement, the astrologer had predicted that this person, whose name they had hidden from him, will have to be hospitalized for the treatment of cancer. My cousins were speechless.

And then they asked, 'Is there a way we can save her? She is our cousin Manisha Koirala.'

The learned man advised that they immediately perform the Mahamrityunjaya puja—or the 'death-conquering ceremony'—followed by havan.

The same day, around fifteen Brahmin priests, wearing thin white linen, duly arrived to perform the ultimate puja to defeat death. They performed their rituals one by one, impressing us with how systematic and coordinated they were. They chanted Lord Shiva's Mahamrityunjaya Mantra 1,00,000 times using the *japa mala*, which is made of 108 beads, offered flowers to the Shiva linga and performed abhisheka with milk and water, followed by *sankalp* (pouring water into a pot and asking for Lord Shiva's blessings). They offered incense, water, *bel* leaves and fruits to the lord. The elaborate ritual came to an end with a massive havan. Our home was filled with sweet-smelling smoke.

The origin of the Mahamrityunjaya Mantra dates back to the Rig Veda. It is a blend of three Hindi words—'*maha*' which means great, '*mrityun*' which means death and '*jaya*' which means victory. The Mahamrityunjaya puja is one of the most important Shiva pujas and is believed to have tremendous benefits. It has the ability to lengthen the lifespan of devotees and save them from life-threatening ailments.

Here is the mantra:

Om tryambakam yajamahe sugandhim pusti vardhanam
Urvarukamiva bandhanan mrtyor mukshiya mamritat.

This can be translated as:

Om. We worship and adore you, O three-eyed one, O Shiva. We meditate on the three-eyed reality which permeates and nourishes all like a fragrance.

This powerful chant is hailed by the sages as the heart of the Vedas.

As the fragrance of the puja mingled with each item and wafted towards me, I sat by myself, lost in thought.

I had learnt that our flight to Mumbai was at 4 p.m. the same day. We had been advised to carry the *rudraksha mala* with us for protection.

I was not quite sure what my thoughts at that point were. I was simply doing what my family wanted me to do.

In fact my thoughts were incoherent even to myself. I cast a glance around my beloved Kathmandu family home. It had started falling apart in places. I had just taken on the task of renovating it.

Will I be back to complete the task? Will I be back to see the maddeningly fragrant 'Night Queen' blossom enticingly in my garden once again? Will I be here when the snow on the Himalayas begins to melt? Will I be . . . at all?

There were too many questions. But no answers.

3

Mumbai

'Confusion, when embraced, is the starting point for discovery, direction and decision.'

—Richie Norton

November 2012

A night-time descent into Mumbai, the capital of Maharashtra, is an entrancing experience. The lights inside the aircraft are off and you feel like you are alone—suspended between the sky and earth.

Located on the west coast of India, Mumbai is home to one of the biggest film industries in the world. In this glamorous world of films, popularly called Bollywood, fortunes and reputations have risen to dizzying heights in no time, and also been shattered and smashed overnight.

This is the city that regularly attracts droves of hopeful youngsters, often from smaller towns, their eyes studded with starry dreams of catching that elusive bird of fame, success and wealth. Mumbai is India's Aladdin's magic lamp. Everyone wishes to rub it and get lucky. The genie has bestowed unimaginable boons on many seekers. It has also denied favours to innumerable others, driving them to despair. And yet there's that attraction, that magical pull.

I had come to Mumbai as an actor in 1990 with my mom after being signed by Subhash Ghai-ji of Mukta Arts for my debut film *Saudagar* which released in 1991 and became a top-grosser. I never looked back.

Movies followed in quick succession, some of which were: *Yalgaar* (1992), *1942: A Love Story* (1994), *Akele Hum Akele Tum* (1995), *Bombay* (1995), *Agni Sakshi* (1996), *Khamoshi: The Musical* (1996), *Gupt* (1997), *Dil Se* (1998), *Kachche Dhaage* (1999), *Mann* (1999) and *Hindustan Ki Kasam* (1999).

Much later, when I was working in a movie with Shah Rukh Khan, he told me, 'Manisha, I think you should buy a house in Mumbai so that you can feel at home here.' I had been living in a rented apartment ever since I came to Mumbai. I was saving money, though I don't know for what! Shah Rukh told me that if I bought a place of my own, I would feel rooted and not feel like a nomad or wanderer. I smiled, because I knew that no house could really tie me down as I have been an eternal nomad by nature.

Shah Rukh, too, had come to Mumbai from Delhi, the same way I had come from Nepal. I guess deep down, I was feeling a little uprooted. I was working hard, but for the longest time, never really felt like I belonged here.

I decided to follow his advice and in 1999 bought my own house and made Mumbai my home.

Mumbai is a city that never sleeps, a city where the young at heart pack in unimaginably long hours of work and top it up by relaxing and hanging out in its shiny pubs and glittering parties all night long. Mumbai's expansive heart is home to millionaires and the homeless, to gangsters and holy men, to the fisherfolk and the elite, to glamorous film stars and overworked commercial sex workers. Despite the city's chaos, nobody wants to leave. For once you bite into Mumbai's enchanted apple, you cannot stay anywhere else.

A great deal has been written and talked about Mumbai's spirit, and rightly so. With a jack-in-the-box resilience, it bounces back and simply moves on after the worst floods, terrorist attacks and communal violence. Despite its hustle and bustle, you feel invigorated by Mumbai's distinct stamp of electric creativity, youthfulness and vitality. Yes, with its cosmopolitan appeal, the city of dreams makes your heart soar.

This time, however, I did not feel any soaring of the spirit as we descended. My heart was in pain. I was gripped by fear. Mom and I had flown into the city alone. The rest of my family was flying in the next day. For the two of us, this was not simply a flight from point A to point B. It was traumatic. I was focused only on meeting Dr Suresh Advani, one of India's best-known oncologists, whom I had set up a consultation with on phone. We were two frightened women trying very hard to come to terms with my condition.

In the aircraft, I had noticed people staring at me. Some in horror, others in sympathy.

How did they know my dark secret?

I felt unnerved by their unrelenting stares. I could feel my mom sitting beside me and grieving silently. I felt bad for her. It was not in divine order that a child should die before her mother.

The darkness of my fear was seeping into my bones now. But I did not want us to become a public spectacle. So I looked at her pale face and wrapped her in her favourite sky blue shawl that I had bought for her on one of my outdoor shoots. Today, after praying for my well-being, she had instinctively brought it along.

I was wearing a grey Juicy Couture tracksuit. To camouflage my bloated stomach I had worn my track pants below my waist. Although, to the casual onlooker, I appeared to be in control, I was not. My hands and legs were trembling. All I wanted was this flight to land soon so that I could get to Dr Advani fast.

As Dr Advani worked elsewhere during the day, he had asked me to meet him at Jaslok Hospital that very evening. I have trusted him implicitly over the years, sending many impoverished Nepali children with cancer to him. He looked after all my patients with the same concern he showed towards the rich and famous. Now I was going to be his patient.

Restlessly, I pulled my cap down and covered the rest of it with my outsized sunglasses. *Why is everything happening so slowly? When will we reach Mumbai?* My heart in my mouth, I surrendered weakly to the knowing gazes around me.

I had not even noticed the stewardess who came and stood next to me, trying to offer me food. I shook my head instinctively. Then another stewardess came, offering me some drinks. I refused. She looked at me compassionately. *Did they too know? Is this why they were being so kind to me?*

The stares followed me even after we landed, or so I thought.

Thankfully, a knot of efficient Airport Authority men met us at the immigration. Swiftly, they guided us into the VIP section and without much delay whisked us out of the airport.

Two things hit me instantly: Mumbai's warm humidity and its distinct smell. I remember many years ago, when I had visited Mumbai as a sixteen-year-old schoolgirl, I had wrinkled my little nose at its fishy smell.

I did not know why that memory came to my mind at that particular time, but it did. Many years of living there had made me become used to Mumbai's salt-in-the-air, fishy smell. But in my Versova home, which is very close to the fishermen's colony, I make it a point to surround myself with a lot of sweet-scented candles, incense and fragrance diffusers. At that point, however, the fear of my diagnosis overwhelmed me. I could hear my heart hammering and feel myself suddenly breaking out into a sweat. My mother was trembling. I caught her arm firmly and whispered, 'Be strong, Ama!' But my voice came out hesitant and weak.

An ambulance was waiting for us at the airport to take us to Jaslok Hospital. Ignoring it, I slid into my own car. When everything in my life was slipping away into unfamiliarity, I needed the security of the familiar. I sank into the comfort of the upholstered leather seat, rested my head on the multiflowered neck pillow which I always keep in my car and took a deep breath.

As we drove towards Jaslok, I felt a rush of fresh panic. I was in a hurry to reach the doctor but found our car caught in bumper-to-bumper traffic. I felt trapped by the private cars, taxis, autorickshaws, buses and trucks around us that were going wild with impatience. Autorickshaws cut lanes while pedestrians tried to cross the streets. People were honking, shouting profanities and threatening each other with dire consequences. Pot-holed roads had been dug up for sewage lines and metro construction, resulting in a huge traffic snarl.

I was bathed in sweat. Anxiety and impatience make a bad cocktail. I wished we had wings. We moved at a snail's pace and, in places, did not move at all. Chaos reigned supreme at points where vehicles were parking illegally, leaving very little space for cars to move.

I twiddled my thumbs in agony and anxiety, feeling suffocated. For an eighteen-kilometre drive that should have taken us twenty-one minutes, it took us a full hour and a half.

* * *

Jaslok Hospital at Pedder Road, south Mumbai, is an imposing grey structure, with bands of light yellow running down from the top. Any other time I would have loved to look at it, located strategically on the main road overlooking the azure expanse of the Arabian Sea and standing tall above the chaos of Mumbai's traffic and numerous billboards.

But my focus this time was on my own health. I was here to meet Dr Advani and felt certain that he would calm my frayed nerves and deal with the issue in the best possible way.

Dr Advani's story has never failed to inspire me. Struck by polio at the age of eight, he had been confined to a wheelchair because of paralysed lower limbs. But his spirit remained undaunted. He was even initially refused admission to medical college because he was 'crippled'. In the early seventies, he selected a field considered not good enough for pursuing—oncology. He then went abroad to train with the best of doctors and came back to India to create innumerable success stories. With sheer hard work and a deep understanding of his field, he emerged as one of the top oncologists in the country and was even bestowed the Padma Bhushan, the country's third-highest civilian award. His contributions are immense and I deeply pray to god that he be bestowed with many such awards in the future.

As soon as we reached the hospital, I jumped out of the vehicle and rushed towards Dr Advani's cabin. In our over-eagerness to meet him, we had arrived earlier than our scheduled time. I was surprised that we had made it, despite the obstacle race our car had been through. Once inside the cabin, I collapsed with exhaustion on the chair. My intense anxiety was also laced with hope. Having faced personal pain himself, Dr Advani would surely know how to deal with my perplexing diagnosis, I thought.

It turned out to be a one-hour wait for the doctor. Mom and I sat in his cabin quietly. There was a hollow feeling in the pit of my stomach. Inside the minimalistic cabin, with its certificate and award-lined walls, I noticed a heart-warming picture of the doctor's family.

And then I saw that my friend Anupama and her husband, Avinash, had arrived. I was so relieved to see them. I have always felt secure in their presence, as if I am being held in somebody's arms and told, 'It's all going to be okay. Don't worry.' They are both caring and dependable.

A thought struck me: *Their marriage appears to be like a fairy tale. But do fairy tales happen in real life?*

My friendship with Anupama is as old as my relationship with Mumbai city. I met this gorgeous, intelligent and funny woman for the first time at Birju Maharaj-ji's kathak class. Anu was training under him as she aspired to be an actress. I was there because Subhash Ghai-ji had signed me and Vivek Mushran for *Saudagar*. I had to learn kathak for the role, while Vivek had to undergo stunt training with the Varma Brothers. Raveena Tandon too was in our batch.

For a long time, Anu and I hardly spoke to each other, but when we did, we instantly bonded and became fast friends. And that's how it has been for the last 20–25 years. She is like a sister to me now.

Avinash belongs to the illustrious Adik family. Anu and Avinash have now been married for sixteen years and have two wonderful sons. Avi is this tall, caring man who knows exactly what to do in a crisis. He brings the word 'super' to my mind. He is super intelligent, super solid and super helpful. Together, Anu and Avi are my beloved extended family.

Avinash is like a son to Mom. They get along really well. I could see how relieved she was too to see him. She instantly held his hand and took him out of the cabin. After explaining everything to him, she entrusted him with the task of finding the best ovarian cancer surgeons in Mumbai. Dr Advani was undoubtedly the best oncologist. But we needed a surgeon.

I have always felt that my mom is an unstoppable, powerful force of nature, especially when it concerns the welfare of her children. Although she appears gentle, she is used to being in control and more often than not, does the right thing. She hurls herself into the task at hand wholeheartedly. Avinash's arrival got her a chance to get back 'into action' instead of waiting endlessly for Dr Advani, while our tension continued to mount.

Alone with Anu now, I let down my guard. Mom was not around. I could finally be myself. I had a meltdown. I caught hold of Anu's shoulders and let the flood from my eyes pour out.

'I don't want to die!' I sobbed.

She hugged and patted my back lovingly. For someone like me who is very private and trained to be in control, this was a difficult moment. I was expressing my deepest fear. But I knew she would understand. After all, she was a mother and a wife. Her eyes showed she understood, and I was grateful.

It was a dark, moonless night. Nothing stirred. I do not like this mood of the day. It depresses me. *When will he arrive?*

Finally, I heard the rolling of a wheelchair in the hospital's long, disinfected corridor and knew that it was Dr Advani. He was wearing a blue striped shirt and loose, khaki trousers.

Below his sparse white hair was perched his square, rimless spectacles. On his lips, he wore a confident smile. After a few pleasantries, I eagerly—rather hurriedly—handed over my reports to him. As he went through them, I tried to read his reaction from his eyes.

We had reached the hospital late in the evening. It was almost 11 p.m. now.

'Well,' he looked up at me with his piercing eyes. 'Manisha, I would like to do another round of tests: PET scans and CT scans. But it's late now. Go home. Come back tomorrow on an empty stomach.'

Dr Advani will do the tests tomorrow and tell me that these reports are inaccurate. I know he will say it's nothing. I can't wait to go back tomorrow morning!

I felt sure that Mom was also thinking that he would tell us that I had been misdiagnosed. I felt hopeful. On our way back, I impulsively asked the driver to stop at the shop that overlooks one of the most recognizable landmarks of Mumbai—Haji Ali. Located on an islet off the coast of Worli in the southern part of Mumbai, Haji Ali Dargah is a mosque and tomb where people of all faiths and religions come to seek blessings. Silently and deeply, we prayed to the saint for my health and well-being.

Haji Ali Juice Centre is one of the city's iconic eating joints and people flock to it between 5 a.m. and 1 a.m. I ordered my favourite—a sitaphal (custard apple) cream. We relished it quietly on our way home.

My Mumbai home. Within its safe space, I have led out my life, with all its ups and downs. On the ground floor, four coveted 'black ladies'—my Filmfare Awards—stand proudly on the dark mahogany round table on the left, next to the white L-shaped sofas. The bright-coloured cushions overlook a wall full of the honours and accolades I have received for my films. This is my public persona—the ornate lamps, the glittering chandeliers.

On the right is a wooden staircase with about twenty steps. It spirals up daintily and leads me to my secluded space—my room. Here I become the real me, minus the frills. My personal space is pretty, quiet, reflective and extremely peaceful. It is my private sanctuary, where I escape from the realities of the world. I love my universe.

I was in a happy mood at this point. Hope seemed a tantalizing possibility.

I cuddled my two beloved dogs, Buddy and Sparky. Sparky was a Pekinese, a tiny white ball of fluffy hair. He was exceptionally temperamental, sensitive and loyal. He melted my heart each time he looked into my eyes with so much love, as if he understood my soul. We had named him Sparky because he had a lot of spark in him. He was a bundle of joy. His death a few years ago broke my heart.

Buddy was a golden retriever, gifted to me as a small puppy around the time of my diagnosis. When I discovered that my treatment would take long, I realized I would not be able to take good care of him. With a heavy heart I gave him away. I had a hard time controlling my tears, but I knew I was doing it with his best interest in mind. It gives me so much happiness to learn today that my Buddy is thriving in his new home.

Delighted to have me home once again, both my pets jumped up at me, vying for attention. I noticed how small Buddy was. He followed me around, though his legs were still not strong enough, and kept wagging his tiny tail. I felt a rush of love for him.

That day, I was convinced that canines have a sixth sense. From the moment I walked in, Buddy became my shadow. He refused to leave me alone even for a second. He followed me wherever I went. He firmly perched himself near my feet and refused to leave. He looked at me with his clear, liquid eyes, as if he wanted to console me. *Could he sense what was in store for me?*

***

As soon as morning dawned, I was up, eager to go to Jaslok and finish off whatever needed to be done. I couldn't wait to restart my normal life which had suddenly been put on pause.

My mother was with me at Jaslok. So was Avinash, along with some other friends of mine. My dad and brother were scheduled to fly in that day and join us directly at the hospital. Tests and scans done, I was asked to check into the hospital room at the end of a long corridor. I was grateful for the privacy it gave me. It was a minimalistic room, sans any decoration. To my right was a window with blinds. My senses were assailed by the typical hospital smell of iodoform.

Once again the long wait for the test results began. I twiddled my thumbs. I fooled around with my mobile phone. I scripted what I would say to the doctor, for I felt certain that he would come and give me the good news that it was a huge mistake.

But time refused to pass quickly. Several hours rolled by—hours in which I kept peeping out into the corridor to check if the doctor was there. It was now beyond lunch time. I was restless, impatient and ready to run all the way up to his cabin.

Around 2 p.m., I heard his wheelchair rolling into the corridor outside my room. Eagerly, I stepped out and looked at him with an expectant smile. My heart missed a beat at his expression. His face was grim, his eyes veiled. *What was happening?*

By this time, many other doctors had trooped in. Avinash
had contacted them for their expert opinion.

I was lying on my back, my stomach protruding. Dr Advani,
along with two or three other accomplished doctors, surrounded
me, looking down at me as if I were a specimen.

It was Dr Advani who spoke directly to me, 'Manisha, it
does appear you have cancer. Late-stage ovarian cancer.'

My world fell apart. But I was not letting this moment go
without asking enough questions to understand things properly.

'So what do we do now?' I asked the group of doctors
around me. It was a clinical, rather than emotional, question.
I had become my practical self now.

One stout doctor with a moustache said, 'I do not
think immediate surgery is the best option. The cancer has
intertwined with her organs.' He looked at the others to make
his point.

I looked on in shock at Dr Advani's crestfallen face and
asked, 'Doctor, what do we do now?' Before he could speak,
another doctor—lean, tall and serious—spoke up, 'It's better
we give her three rounds of chemotherapy, shrink the tumour,
perform the operation and then give her another three rounds
of chemo to complete the process.'

I asked Dr Advani, 'Doctor, what do you say? Don't you
think that the normal procedure is the best? Surgery first and
then chemo?'

He remained deep in thought, as if he were weighing the
options. And then he looked directly at me and said, 'Perhaps.
But you see, the cancer has intertwined with your organs, so . . .'
Another doctor completed the sentence, 'It's risky. And very
complicated.'

I was in an argumentative mode. Like a recalcitrant child,
I asked, 'What if after the operation, some cancer cells are left

behind? Will the chemo destroy all of it? What will happen if some cancer cells refuse to get destroyed? What then?'

A cloud of worry seemed to drop over Dr Advani's eyes. I looked around. That same expression seemed to be reflected in the eyes of all the doctors in the room. I turned my head away towards the window with its view of the Arabian Sea outside. I was struggling to fight my terror. I pushed my nails into the palm of my hands. It hurt, but not so much as the pain of disappointment in my heart.

Outside the room, my mom was in full action mode. She was making one call after another. There was a flurry of activity. My friend, Paulomi Sanghavi, too, had arrived by then.

Paulomi and I became friends around fifteen years ago. She is my closest girlfriend. We have travelled to many countries together and shared many happy times—shopping, going to restaurants, laughing at silly things and generally enjoying ourselves. A strong-headed Gujarati woman from a family that owns several huge factories and is in the business of importing and exporting clothing, she asserted her individuality by not joining the family business and becoming a jeweller instead. She now has a dazzling designer store in Mumbai's Hughes Road. Fashionable and practical, Paulomi is a strong, independent woman who has seen me through my best phase as well as my worst. She always knows the right thing to do.

Assessing the grimness of the situation, Paulomi immediately called up her sister, Dr Premal, an oncosurgeon based in Virginia, USA. As she spoke on the phone, she kept nodding vigorously. She seemed to agree with her sister that I should be flown to the US immediately for treatment. There was a garble of voices outside. Paulomi's self-assured voice intermingled with my mother's nervous one. Mom was busy reaching out to all her friends in the US. She has a host of girlfriends across the country, all of them senior scientists and doctors in top hospitals.

My dad and Bhai too had arrived by then. Later, my brother told me about how angry he had been on witnessing the chaos around this sudden decision to take me to the US. He had heard Paulomi talking to her sister in the US and Mom speaking to Mukul Aunty and Meena Aunty and her other friends there. He felt strongly that my entire support system—my home, my friends, his own friends—were in India. This sudden decision to take me to the US agitated him. He also felt nervous and unsure about how he would manage in New York—a place he knew nothing about. He was upset with all of us.

I had zoned out completely. All I could think of was going along with everybody's decision. All the doctors here were telling me it was a very complicated case. So why should I risk my life by not going to the best place in the world? When everyone around informed me that we would leave for America, I simply nodded. I was too weary to think. I could not make any more decisions.

Another fear resurfaced at that very moment. If we did go to the US for treatment, where would we stay? And for how long? I knew many people in America and had several friends there. In fact, many of them had even lovingly invited me over to their homes whenever I visited. But this was different. I was not a glamorous movie star; I was a cancer patient. Who would want me in their home? My heart sank. Instantly, my mind flew to the time I had offered my Mumbai home to a family from Nepal who had come for their son's treatment at Tata Memorial Hospital, Mumbai. But how could I expect the same gesture from anyone? It was not fair.

Okay, I would need money. Lots of it. I called up my financial adviser, Mona, and got busy asking her details of how much investment I had in bonds and shares. 'Liquidate everything!' I instructed. But my heart knew that even that might not be enough. How could the rupee stand up against the strong US dollar? How would it suffice for our extended stay in New York?

Paulomi was at her best in this crisis. She got busy calculating the funds I had and told me roughly how much the treatment abroad would cost. I looked at her in horror.

And then she said something I did not expect to hear, 'Manisha, please call up Sahara Shree and tell him your situation. He has a hotel in New York. Just ask him for help.'

I was horrified. I have always been shy and reserved about asking for favours. But after a lot of deliberation and gathering tremendous courage, I decided to call up Subrata Roy, fondly called Sahara Shree. Roy is the managing worker and chairman of Sahara India Pariwar, an Indian conglomerate with diversified businesses and ownership interests that include New York's Plaza Hotel.

I had met him several times at business events with other celebrities and developed a deep respect for him. I was impressed by his humanitarian spirit, especially his efforts to provide financial support to the families of the 127 Kargil martyrs. I had never imagined that I would be in a position where I would have to ask him for help. I was embarrassed and did not know what his response would be. But I also knew deep inside that without this help, we would not be able to last many days in New York.

With trembling hands, I dialled his number. I shall never forget his response. He was warm, genuinely concerned and eager to help, given my situation. His words were music to my ears. Not only did he ask us to stay at his hotel but also told me that he knew a few people there who could assist us were we to need any help. I was overwhelmed. I learnt later that Sahara Shree used to call up my doctors and keep a tab on my progress.

I do not know how politically correct it is to mention him today, knowing how events unfolded adversely for him later on, but my family and I will always remain indebted to him for his generosity at a time we needed it most.

The days ahead were a blur. All I knew was that we were soon heading to the US. They were all determined to go. My parents and my brother.

In hindsight, I laugh when I recall the situation. So consumed were we with the end result of reaching America—to somehow bring me back to health—that we forgot to consider the most important detail. Going to America would require a visa! It suddenly dawned on my family that none of them except me possessed that precious stamp. They looked at each other in dismay.

Would that mean I would have to fly alone? They shook their heads in unison, determined not to allow such a preposterous thing to happen. My family is quite cute that way—they are my dependable army, but ever so often forget to carry their weapons to a war!

Thankfully, luck favoured us. The US embassies of both India and Nepal helped us in getting our visas quickly. So now, the date for our departure was set—1 December 2012—exactly four days after we landed in Mumbai.

In the days that followed, I found my heart expanding. My reports had not come out the way I had expected them to. I felt myself opening up to the wisdom around me. I listened to everyone who cared to give me advice. I was a flower, my petals open, soaking in the sun.

While inside my home, I preferred to stay in my sanctuary upstairs, immersed in a roller coaster of emotions. I could sense that the rooms downstairs were filled with people. Relatives and well-meaning friends had flocked to meet me. But I preferred to be left alone.

My trance was broken as soon as I heard the sound of someone coming up the wooden stairs. I looked up. It was Zakia, the fashion photographer. I had met her a few times at Deepti Naval's home. Zakia had called me up to ask whether she could come over and I had said yes.

Zakia is an attractive and stylish woman. She has a great sense of fashion, which is natural, considering the profession she is in.

She came up to my bedroom. She spoke softly, unlike many others who were throwing around loud advice of all sorts. Perhaps seeing a cancer patient in the family sensitizes one to the feelings of others and makes one more respectful of another person's private space.

Sheepishly, she asked me, 'Manisha, may I share something with you?'

'Of course!' I said, knowing that her words were born out of affection and concern for me.

I welcomed these comments as much as I detested the frivolity of those sympathizers who said to me: 'You'll be fine!' or worse, 'Probably you do not have cancer at all.'

I was no fool. I knew that the doctors at Kathmandu and Mumbai were not hoodwinking me. Yes, I did have cancer.

So here was Zakia giving me precious tips from the learnings culled from her sister's three-time cancer relapse.

'And she is still alive after twenty-five years, Manisha.' That was just the morale booster I needed.

You mean cancer patients could last twenty-five years after treatment? Not bad. Not bad at all!

So I listened to Zakia's wise tips carefully and kept them close to my heart. This is what she told me:

- There are new treatment methods available for cancer. It can be treated efficiently.
- During chemotherapy, tell yourself that these are vitamin shots that will destroy each cancer cell in your body.
- Eat healthy and nutritious food to keep your immune system strong.
- Slow-cook vegetables of five colours in a lentil soup and drink this rainbow.
- Drink lots of water to wash away the toxins.

And then she did the sweetest thing possible. She handed me her warm black Burberry jacket. 'You can give it back to me when you return.' My heart soared.

She is confident that I will live long enough to come back and return her jacket? Yay! Can I give living a try?

I wore that jacket lovingly. It reminded me of the selfless girl who kept in touch with me on Skype and never once burdened me with the huge family problems she was facing back then. I will always be grateful to my friends for supporting me empathetically.

I finally accepted that I had cancer. The rancorous information seeped into me drop by drop like a bitter medicine. It shook me rudely awake from my stupor of denial. I became very pensive and quiet.

I remember, on the last day of my departure, I got this sudden urge to see Mumbai in all its glory and chaos, as if to capture the images in my heart. I set off in my car, asking the driver to take me towards south Mumbai.

I wanted to see the magnificence of the island, the majesty of the skyscrapers and the tenacity of the have-nots. I love the sea. I love its confident girth, its benevolent expanse. I love the way Marine Drive's promenade embraces the sapphire Arabian Sea. During the day, the waters glisten under the sun. Viewed at night from an elevation, Marine Drive turns into a string of glittering pearls. No wonder it is known as the Queen's Necklace.

It was a bright sunny morning. The traffic at this hour was disciplined, not chaotic. It was a beautiful, peaceful sight. I rolled my windows down and breathed in the tangy air. A gentle breeze ruffled my hair and my tongue tasted salt.

As my driver drove past Chowpatty Beach, one of the famous public beaches adjoining Marine Drive in the Girgaon area of Mumbai, I saw flocks of white seagulls on the beach. It was a sight I can never forget. Everywhere I looked, there were these majestic birds, spreading their wings and fluttering around. Their harsh wailing and squeaking calls filled the air. Mesmerized, I asked my driver to stop the car.

I had read somewhere that these migratory birds come to Mumbai between October and March in search of warmer climes. A random thought struck me. The birds had travelled thousands of miles, crossing continents, to escape the winter there. And I? I was travelling away from the warmth of my Mumbai into the cold of America. It made for a beautiful thought and I almost smiled.

Just then, a regal white seagull broke away from the flock and came quite close to us. I was fascinated by the black markings on its head and wings as well as the perfection of its webbed orange feet. Suddenly, before my horrified eyes, it swooped down and caught an unsuspecting little bird in its stout, longish bill. I could not see what bird it was, but it was small, feathery and helpless.

Little bird, fight! Don't give up so easily!

As if on cue, the little bird began struggling. Furiously.

The sight saddened me. Here was this innocent bird bobbing about in the seashore, enjoying the sunny day. Little did it know what destiny had in store for her.

I looked up at the blue sky. My eyes were blinded by the sun. The determined seagull had flown away. The unpredictability of life hit me forcefully.

I felt unhappy. Life was so fragile.

Who will win? The prey or the predator? I do not know. And perhaps never will.

4

New York

'For life and death are one, even as the river and the sea are one.'
                                                                 —*Kahlil Gibran*

December 2012

It was a crisp winter day in New York. I was in a rush to deplane the moment our Air India flight touched down at LaGuardia airport. My heart was beating fast. I was getting closer to my goal of availing what I hoped was the best medical cure. I could not wait to meet my doctor. Two old friends, Vicky and Yasir, along with a few people who worked for Sahara Shree, were there to receive us. I was happy to see Chetna Di, my father's only sister, and Praveen Da, her husband.

As we stepped out of the airport, I could feel my lungs perk up with the freshness of the winter air. My cheeks and nose started tingling. I braced myself to face the cold. Quickly, we got into a taxi and began cruising along to Plaza Hotel.

In many ways, New York reminded me of Mumbai. Like Mumbai, this too is a city that never sleeps. But if Mumbai is Windows version 2.0, New York is Windows version 10.

New York is like a huge heart—ever pulsating, ever throbbing. The constant flow of people is like the complex network of arteries and blood vessels—ever moving, never stopping. With its magnificent Broadway shows, multiculturalism and high fashion, New York is the circulatory pump that to me is the centre of the world.

But all that vitality around me served only to stab my heart about my lack of it at this point. As we drove along, I was struck by the dominant colour of black worn by fashionable New Yorkers.

In my current frame of mind, however, I could not appreciate the city's appeal.

Then suddenly, our car passed over East River on to a majestic two-level double-cantilever bridge, with one cantilever span over the channel on each side of Roosevelt Island. This was the historical Queensboro Bridge—the structure about which Nick Carraway from Scott Fitzgerald's classic *The Great Gatsby* famously commented:

> The city seen from the Queensboro Bridge is always the city seen for the first time, in its first wild promise of all the mystery and the beauty in the world.

Our driver was in a chatty mood. He informed us that the bridge did not have suspended spans, so each of the cantilever arms reached till the middle. For a long time, this had been the longest cantilever span in North America, bridging Manhattan and Roosevelt Island, until Quebec Bridge, built in 1917, surpassed it.

I was barely listening. My eyes fell sightlessly on the expanse of the East River as it whizzed past my window. The New York skyline reached out to the sky and I became lost in thought.

This was not my first visit to the city. I had come here in 1993 as part of a film troupe. We were on our last leg of the tour, after performing around twenty shows in the UK and various cities of the US. In our troupe were actors like Aamir Khan, Salman Khan, Pooja Bhatt and Shilpa Shetty. At the New York show, Amitabh Bachchan-ji and Juhi Chawla too joined us. We performed there at a huge auditorium in front of a cheering audience of over 25,000. Then, in 2004, I spent many months at New York University, studying film-making. I was also trying to get a feel of the city to decide whether I could live there.

The first visit is as difficult to forget as first love. I had passed through this same bridge in 1993 to reach Manhattan. Suddenly, I was overcome with a strange feeling—the abrupt lifting of a curtain from a hoary past. It was as if I had passed through several consecutive doorways and emerged from an ancient one.

A strong feeling of déjà vu consumed me—as if I had lived here. How, when, where—I did not know. Yet the certainty of this recollection was as clear as my sitting in this cab right now. Shadowy memories of shared togetherness, laughter, love and the sudden pain of parting—of leaving a previous body—nudged at my soul. Piercing through the misty curtain of time emerged a hazy memory of having lived and died in this city in another lifetime.

Why was I feeling the same way now? Yes, I had definitely made this city my home before. *Yes, this would be a good city to die in . . . yet again.*

I kept mulling over thoughts of death. I just could not shake off the feeling. It was a numbness born out of a terror of the nameless.

And suddenly we were there. Before me stood the twenty-storey luxury landmark hotel at Midtown Manhattan. As we entered the main entrance at 768 Fifth Avenue, I felt dwarfed by its opulence and grandeur. Nothing I had seen before matched its magnificence.

Despite the terror my body was nurturing, I stopped to let it all sink in. This was the place where the Beatles had stayed in 1964, where famous performers and internationally known singers had left their mark and where Donald Trump had wed Marla Maples in a grand ceremony with 1500 invited guests.

All my life, I had been fascinated by stories around the goings-on at the Palm Court, the Champagne Bar, the Edwardian Room, the Terrace Room, the Rose Club, the Grand Ball Room and the Plaza Food Hall. An avid follower of Hollywood movies, I had excitedly watched scenes shot in this hotel in some of my favourite films: *North by Northwest, Funny Girl, Plaza Suite, Scent of a Woman, Sleepless in Seattle* and *Home Alone 2: Lost in New York.*

The lavishness of the hotel was enhanced by the festivity of Christmas. The glow of lights on the huge tree that reached the magnificent ceiling illuminated the entire hall, lending it a golden sheen. It was other-worldly.

I looked around quietly at all the fashionable people. I could hear the click-clack of skyscraper heels on the shiny floors and the dignified shuffle of coats and briefcases. People went about their business in a quiet, composed manner. I was certain they led shiny, glossy lives. My heart scrunched at what had just happened to mine.

A pretty woman with sky-blue eyes was holding the hand of the cutest toddler I had ever seen. She came up to me, dropped her gaze on my huge belly and smiled in the conspiratorial manner only a woman who has gone through the same experience can give a seemingly pregnant one.

No, no, it's not a pregnancy. You have a baby already! What would you know of the misery of one who wants to, but can't?

With apologies to those women who do not agree with me on this issue, I want to express myself freely here. I feel that the biggest gift nature has given a woman is that of motherhood. I feel that becoming a mother brings a woman into full bloom and is one of the biggest assets she can possess.

Secretly, I have always wanted to have babies of my own. I have been driven by this thought. I have wanted to have a home, family and husband. What I have desperately wanted, however, has been to have babies of my own. But I guess it was not meant to be.

Even now, after being cancer-free, I long to adopt a baby but am nervous. I wonder whether with my high levels of stress I would be able to do justice to my role as a mother.

Misery mixed with guilt as I stroked my protruding abdomen. To the onlooker, I appeared to be nine months pregnant. Nothing could be more untrue.

Inside my belly was a whole murky, dark kingdom where a grand conspiracy of unimaginable scale was being planned. The treacherous enemy had stealthily invaded my body and reproduced its tribe until it was swelling and ready to break free of its confines. A takeover plan was about to be executed in the dimness within. The shadowy enemy was scheming about how and when to obliterate the host—me.

I remained pensive as the butler showed us to our rooms. My mind did register how impressive the room was, but my heart was too heavy to notice the details. My eyes were too tired to be appreciative.

Yet, for a brief moment, my mind wavered.

What a lovely setting this would be to die in! It would be a grand exit, enjoying five-star luxuries and the services of these regal butlers!

Instantly, however, the absurdity of the thought made me dismiss it. Death was simply not acceptable.

Quietly, each of us dispersed to our rooms—Mom and Dad in one, my brother Siddharth and Biru (a family friend from Delhi) in another and Paulomi and I in the third. Stepping quietly into our room, I shut the door tight.

Finally, I was with my thoughts. My brain felt woozy due to the jet lag. My body ached. Every cell of my body seemed aware that it was under attack from a powerful enemy.

I almost felt sorry for it. As I am used to doing in the hour of crisis, I decided to act. My shy personality underwent a change. I now wanted to reach out to people who could possibly help me. Perhaps I was scared to deal with my thoughts alone. I needed something positive to hang on to—like a lifeline.

I sat cross-legged on the huge downy bed and sank into its comfort. I began typing emails.

The first one was to Dr Narayan Naidu whom I was introduced to by my holistic healer, Irma, in Mumbai. She had suggested that Dr Naidu could be of some help if I ever needed him. In a frenzy, I sent another email to Mom Luang, the Princess of Thailand, whom I had met sometime back. She had casually told me then of a naturopathic doctor who had cured somebody's cancer. I also shot off a few emails to some friends, asking for their advice. Perhaps they might have heard of some other successful therapies?

I realized that I was flying off into unknown territory, but I reasoned with myself that this was the best strategy. If these were to be my last days on earth, I might as well give my all to trying out every possible option.

Now that I had completed every task I could think of, I was once again alone with my thoughts. To avoid thinking too deeply, I strolled out of the room and looked down at the luxurious lobby.

Once again, everything and everyone seemed wrapped in happiness. People were laughing, kissing and cuddling. They were celebrating life. And here I was—a miserable patient, fighting to be alive.

The thought of leaving such a beautiful world behind depressed me further. In the adjoining room, I heard sounds of Ama weeping. She was talking to her friends on the phone and trying to find comfort in their advice. A wave of guilt swept over me.

Conflicting emotions ran through me. I should have been protecting her in her old age instead of inflicting pain on her. How could I put her through this trauma?

Despair made me head to the bathroom. In the solitude of the marbled floor and the gold-plated fittings, the reality and the magnitude of my grief hit me.

Under normal circumstances, I would have got a bubbly tub ready and soaked in the scented oil and bath salts. That was the way I soothed and calmed my frayed nerves. This time, however, it was different. I looked down at myself in distaste. I had begun to feel my body did not belong to me. I was a caricature of what I once was. Where was my slim waist? Where had this protrusion come from? I simply turned on the shower and let the cold water hit my head in full force.

Without warning, a guttural cry rose from deep within me. The tears tumbled out in a storm—until my whole body was shaking and my brain felt tattered from inside. The loneliness of dying seemed frightening. It was the kind of loneliness that corroded my insides.

I wept in empathy for my parents. For the grief they would feel after losing their child. I joined them in their mourning for me. I cried for every mother who had lost her precious child. I cried for every young life that had been cut short. I cried for myself.

As the water kept pounding me, my shoulders began to shake uncontrollably. Contorted by the onslaught of primal emotions, my heart felt hollow. And yet the tears would not stop.

This was the first time I actually cried since my diagnosis. Earlier, I was either in denial or conscious of revealing my true feelings to my mother. But now, underneath the furious, relentless assault of the water from the shower, I finally felt safe. I could be myself.

What had the great performer Charlie Chaplin once said? 'I always like walking in the rain, so no one can see me crying.'

How had he voiced my deepest emotions?

I think my weeping bout continued forever. Soon, my breathing became ragged and I began gasping for breath.

I felt sure that the enormity of my grief and its intensity had disintegrated bits of my soul and made it run out on to the marbled floor, forming a private black lake of grief. The blackness must now be running into the crevices, looking for an escape.

Sorrow, regret, gloom, dejection and heartache mixed with despondency, suffering, anguish and heart-wrenching wails to form a dark mix of slush, sludge, muck. I could feel this thick black liquid clogging the pipes and running feverishly into the hotel's sewage system. I could feel it sliding forward with purpose until it reached the ceiling of the grand hall. Had the heavy, oil-laden dark drops seeped through the grand carpets and begun dripping messily on to the decorated Christmas tree and the shining floors? Was it making people slip on its squishy sliminess?

It was an ugly thought. And frightening.

My feet were trembling and ready to give way. My hands shuddering, I turned the shower off and dried myself—including my disobedient middle section of the body.

I felt spent and exhausted. Much like a sack that had suddenly collapsed after its contents were emptied.

Unknown to me, a major shift had taken place inside me. The tears had cleared away a lot of clutter. It suddenly dawned on me that acceptance had finally seeped in. And with that was born a brave strategy.

I would now send my soldiers into the depths of the mysterious shadowy kingdom festering inside my stomach. They would put up a resistance. And, if need be, go down fighting.

No longer will I remain a passive observer. I will now become an active participant in my treatment, I decided.

5

Meeting Dr Chi

'Hope is being able to see that there is light despite all of the darkness.'
                                                                —*Desmond Tutu*

4 December 2012

After a nail-biting wait of three days we finally got to meet Dr Dennis Chi, head, section of ovarian cancer surgery, Memorial Sloan Kettering Cancer Center (MSKCC)—an impressive white-and-sky-blue building with the American flag fluttering proudly atop it. Founded in 1884 as the New York Cancer Hospital, the MSKCC is the largest and oldest private cancer centre in the world with inspiring success stories.

We had heard that Dr Chi was an extremely busy man, that his calendar was always full. Luckily, we got an appointment through the intervention of my mom's school friend Meena Aunty, whom she knew from her Benares days. Her husband, Dr Jhanawar, was working then in the administration department of Sloan Kettering. On my mom's request he had been kind enough to help us get an earlier appointment. Had it not been for Dr Jhanawar, we would never have been able to meet the extremely busy Dr Chi so soon.

Dr Chi's credentials and 'medical lore' impressed all of us. He had spent over twenty years of his surgical career caring for women with cancerous and non-cancerous gynaecological diseases. He led the field in cutting-edge research, set high standards for state-of-the-art care and had performed many ovarian cancer surgeries successfully.

On googling Dr Chi, I found this on the MSKCC website:

> My mother was an ob-gyn, so I entered my residency thinking I would take over her practice. However, during my first year of training, I was exposed to gynecologic oncology patients and the procedures used to treat cancers. I saw how quality of care and surgery were so essential to good outcomes for these patients. This inspired me to go into the sub specialty of gynecologic oncology. I wanted to develop an expertise in advanced ovarian cancer surgery because I saw that this was the area where training, skill, dedication, and perseverance made the most difference.[1]

I was filled with optimism. So there we were—my closest people and I, buoyed by the confidence-boosting stories about Dr Chi. I sat on the farthest chair in the waiting room, praying that he would give me hope. God knew I badly needed it.

I took quick, light steps into his cabin, positive that he would finally 'fix' my problem. A slice of New York sunlight fell into his cabin from the window to the right.

I have always believed that I have a strong sense of intuition about people. My first feeling on meeting Dr Chi was a sense of relief. I felt splashed with sunshine. Dr Chi is a Korean with Mongolian features, and his eyes speak of confidence.

---

[1] 'Dennis S. Chi, MD, FACOG, FACS', Memorial Sloan Kettering Cancer Center, https://www.mskcc.org/cancer-care/doctors/dennis-chi.

I focused hard on reading his face. I wanted the truth. I tried reading his eyes. *Nothing.* I tried reading his expression. *Nothing.*

His expression didn't give anything away as he looked carefully through my reports. He thumbed each page slowly. I could not take it any more and asked him, 'Dr Chi, have you done this kind of complicated surgery before? I mean, for late-stage ovarian cancer?'

'Yes,' he replied. He didn't look up.

'How long did that patient live?'

'She is alive and doing fine.'

I heaved a sigh of relief.

I felt happy that finally a doctor had agreed with what I had heard was the best protocol—surgery first and six rounds of chemotherapy later. Both Dr Suresh Advani at Jaslok Hospital, Mumbai, and Dr Thomas A. Kaputo at Cornell Hospital, New York, had felt that it should be the other way round—three rounds of chemo first, followed by surgery and then three more rounds of chemo.

I was hoping some doctor would do it the standard way. And here was Dr Chi telling me that this was exactly the protocol he would follow.

Though relieved, I continued to ask more questions, meekly: 'Doctor, will you cut my stomach horizontally or vertically?'

Dr Chi looked up and smiled, 'I know my job. Please don't worry.' He must have met many crazy patients in his career. I was sure he would remember me as one of them.

We Koiralas are very family-centric. We are there for each other in every crisis and this was one of unexpected magnitude. So here we were—my parents, my brother, my close relatives and friends. Looking back, I smile when I think of what onlookers must have thought. An entourage of 10–12 very anxious people moving together in groups, all with similar serious expressions.

But after the meeting, there appeared a hint of a smile on all our faces. Not complete smiles, because we did not dare do that, lest the evil eye cast its glance on us, stalling our dreams. But this time, all of us had a spring in our feet. We left his office quietly, not betraying our real emotions. Once inside my hotel room, we all melted.

Beams of joy flew across the room, bounced off our faces and wrapped us all in a big group-hug of warmth.

This was perhaps the first time we had smiled as a family. Hanging on to that branch of hope, I felt like a little child swinging joyfully on a mango tree. So, it would all turn out fine, after all. Dr Chi had been the first doctor to give me hope. I wanted to hug him with gratitude.

If that patient could live, why couldn't I, I asked myself nonchalantly.

Rumi's beautiful words floated into my mind at that very moment, 'Darkness is your candle. Your boundaries are your quest.'

* * *

Dr Chi had informed us that my surgery would be on 10 December. I wanted to use this time to research about my condition, its prognosis and the alternative treatments available. I was determined to arm myself with information so that I could feel empowered and not helpless. I would also use this time to catch up with Shail Mama who, for me, represented New York.

I sent emails to a few close friends and received warm, loving messages back. I shut my iPad. It felt good to be cared for.

How do you spell hope, I asked my heart? Pat came the reply, 'You don't spell it. You feel it.' That's settled then. I would create my own sunshine . . .

6

Broken, but Picked Up by Love

'Happiness is having a large, loving, caring, close-knit family in another city.'

—George Burns

2–9 December 2012

Chetna Di, my father's only sister, was one of the people who reinforced my belief in the reassuring power of family and friends. We share a mutual fondness for each other and our families are very close.

I had rushed to Virginia to be by her side in January 2012 on learning that she had zero-stage breast cancer. My distress turned to relief when I saw that she was recovering well. However, I could not push away the thought of our family history. I had lost several family members to cancer. Unease and worry raced through me.

Little did I know that by the end of 2012, the tables would get turned. My aunt would be visiting me after my cancer diagnosis.

During my treatment in New York, my uncle, Praveen Da, and Chetna Di went out of their way to take care of us, spending most of their off days with me and my family. They would drive down all the way from Virginia, spend the weekends with us and then drive back to their work.

I will never forget how they made our cold New York winters warm with their love. They brought thoughtful gifts for each one of us, including much-needed winter clothes. For me, Chetna Di would get the softest T-shirts, loose pyjamas (to accommodate my bloated stomach), socks, mufflers and caps. She took great care to ensure that the comfortable clothes she brought for me did not graze my chemotherapy-induced sensitive skin.

Chetna Di also brought clothes for Dad and Mom, as also food items for us. Since our decision to go to the US had been sudden, we were unprepared for a longer stay. So Chetna Di brought familiar utensils that she knew Mom would need for cooking in a new country. Her care and affection and Praveen Da's quirky wit kept us all in good humour.

It is in a crisis such as this that one realizes the value of people who stand by you. Chetna Di and Praveen Da stand tall in this regard.

* * *

Besides them and my immediate family—Mom, Dad and my bhai, Siddharth—there emerged a supportive, affectionate army around me comprising Mridula Di, Mukul Aunty, Dipika Aunty, Meena Aunty, Kumi Aunty, Lulu Rana and Sudhir Vaishnav-ji. I was deeply grateful for their presence and began drawing strength from them.

My entourage remained busy in their own anxious little worlds, all centering around me.

My brother, Biru and Sudhir Vaishnav-ji were constantly in and out of the hospital trying to understand the administrative side of things, working out the cost of treatment, understanding the procedure and the protocol of admitting an international patient, which they discovered was not easy. None of us had any clue. So Bhai became totally engaged in all this.

Chetna Di and Praveen Da busied themselves with thinking of ways to make us comfortable in a country they lived in. Lulu Rana, a survivor of breast cancer herself, brought along a wig for me. Smilingly, she told me that I would need it soon. She prepared me for what lay ahead. Mridula Aunty lovingly got some home-cooked meals for me.

My mother had her family friends who supported her emotionally. Mridula Aunty would be with her whenever she could. Mom also called up her friends and sought blessings from Pilot Baba. While in her own space, she would cry on the phone, asking for blessings and prayers. With me, she remained calm.

Dad dealt with pain in his own way. As he is a very quiet person, he kept his feelings to himself. He is a very sensitive and caring person and does not like being a burden on anyone. My brother noticed that he had fallen very silent and kept reading the same book again and again—often as many as seven to eight times. He would remain engrossed in them. He would get books from people and ask for those on healing. Those were the days Dad discovered Dr Andrew Weil's book on achieving optimum health through the body's natural healing power. He became interested in the field of integrative medicine and the healing-oriented approach to healthcare that encompasses body, mind and spirit. He started reading other books by Dr Weil. I guess this was Dad's way of dealing with the crisis at hand—quietly and in the most dignified way possible.

To tell you the truth, my entourage, though busy, felt clueless and helpless themselves. What they felt they were up against was far too big for them to comprehend or deal with.

My friend Paulomi set aside all her personal work and accompanied me to New York during my most difficult period. She remained with me until the surgery.

Now confidence was a quality I badly needed those days. My self-esteem was at its lowest and I felt useless. I constantly fought swirls of darkness rising within me. It threatened to choke me. It was a feeling I could not share with anyone.

I remember that beautiful morning—just a day before my operation. I had been avoiding people as I was no longer sure of myself. But that day, Paulomi insisted that I go with her to buy something she needed. Reluctantly, I stepped out of the hotel.

Emerging out of the familiar, I suddenly felt overwhelmed at the sheer number of people around me—all striding along energetically. I was amazed by what I saw. Being a woman, and a fashionable one in Bollywood's heydays, I gazed in awe at the fashionable ladies ramp-walking on the streets in their high heels.

Yes, they were all there, mostly turned out in black. To a fashionista like me, New York appeared to be a non-stop high-end fashion parade.

There was the power suit, the structured-jacket-on-the-shoulder look, the leather mini with training sneakers, the sexy shirt with a casual sweatshirt, the jumpsuit with platform heels, the statement leather with boots, the monochrome look with dark shades, the contrast oversized pieces with designer bags, the rugged sneakers and the just-rolled-out-of-bed T-shirt with designer heels.

And as if to rebel against the monotony of the stylish black was the casually elegant multi-coloured look: the cross-body bag with a statement strap, the run-free-in-a-slip dress, the throw-and-go backpack, the all-rocker-grunge look with vintage tees, the undone blazer, the baggy trousers, the parka with a playful dress.

But something strange happened to me while these women were striding forward confidently. My heart began to beat rapidly, my breath began coming out in short puffs, my face burnt with hot flashes and my head suddenly felt very light. Fear gripped me. I began sweating and shaking.

As we entered a sprawling mall, I was overcome by a strong sense of impending doom. It was accompanied by nausea, chest pain, headache, numbness and tingling.

Am I having a heart attack? Am I dying?

Suddenly, Paulomi turned towards me and said, 'My god, sweetie! Are you having a panic attack?'

And then, she soothed and reassured me by saying the sweetest words, 'You are in the best place for your treatment. Don't worry.'

But my shaking just would not stop!

She held my arms protectively and gently walked me back to my hotel room. All the time, she kept on saying, 'It's okay. It's all going to be fine, Manisha!' Gently, she made me lie on my bed, made sure I was covered and warm and left to continue her shopping.

That memory is on top of my list when I think of Paulomi. The compassionate gesture placed her firmly on my heart's Wall of Fame.

* * *

To me New York has always meant Shail Mama. I always associate this dazzling city with him. Shail Upadhya was my mother's cousin, hence my uncle—my *mama*. He was quite a dandy and had introduced me to New York in 1993 and later in 2004 when I had come to the city to study film-making. He is one person whose memory will remain etched in my heart forever.

Mama had quite an illustrious career and we were extremely proud of his achievements. He had come to the US from Nepal as the head of the United Nation's peacekeeping efforts and in this significant role, he had remained in New York from the 1960s to the 1980s.

After his retirement from the United Nations, he lived in a swanky apartment opposite the Shah of Iran's. All the top diplomats lived in that lane. During weekends, he would go to his weekend Southampton home to spend time with his long-term girlfriend, Karen. Though they never married, I think they were closer to each other than any husband and wife. I was greatly distressed when I learnt of her passing. How must he be coping without his beloved by his side, I wondered.

In the middle of my film career, I had flown to this city in 2004. It was a time when I had begun feeling suffocated with my non-stop dress-up-make-up-act-change routine. At one point I was doing twelve films in a year! I had started feeling like a robot who was taken to the most exotic locales and countries, but never got the chance to explore anything beyond the film set.

Being a girl who hailed from a mountainous country, I longed to be close to nature. I wanted to see beaches when it rained, golden sunsets from mountain tops and nature in all its wild glory. I badly wanted to experience real life, meet real people and see all the stunning places we recreated in our movies.

Mama's New York seemed to be the perfect escape. If you ask me the truth, I was actually testing the waters to see if I could shift base here permanently.

Mama was a kind as well as a fun-loving man. He understood my deepest desires. In a wish-granted sort of way, he began taking me to high-end fashion shows, interesting museums, awe-inspiring art exhibitions and the most happening restaurants. He seemed to be on a roll—introducing me to his most fashionable friends and showing me all things wonderful in Manhattan. With him as my beloved guide and companion, I began feeling at home in the city. I remember Karen Aunty helping me choose a very pretty yellow summery dress one morning when Mama was taking me to the races. I think it suited me. I could see it in Mama's eyes.

But it was Mama's unique style of dressing that made him stand out in the crowd. After his retirement, he became a men's clothing designer, catering to the rich and the famous.

I found his fashion sense quite fascinating. He wore black and white all his life. He would match a black-and-white checked shirt with black-and-white striped trousers. Then he would match monochromes with a cap of polka dots and stars. Creating new patterns in black and white was a passion for him—one that he was very proud of. Smugly, he told me once that a top designer had copied his style. The next thing he knew was that black and white had become the newest trend in the designer's collection. He also often talked about his friendship with the famous stylist Donna Karan.

Even though I had laughed about it, I was proud of him for being featured in the documentary *Bill Cunningham New York*. In truth, he had begun getting recognized as a part of New York's fashion scene. He was often photographed in his plaid suits, chequered ties and Warhol blazers for the *New York Times's* style section. I was in awe of him as he flitted from one home to another in New York, Southampton and Miami.

Because of our past bonding, I was in a hurry to meet him this time. Shail Mama had not changed over the years. He was as kind, as warm and as fun-loving as I remembered him.

But my discerning eyes noticed that he had changed after his beloved's death. He had become weak. He needed a stick to walk and even though he did not express it, I could sense the heaviness of his emotional burden.

He had told my mom, 'God cannot be that unkind. He will save Manisha!'

He was very happy to see me and did not hide his pleasure. I had visited his apartment earlier in 1993. I had then wondered what a black-and-white apartment would look like! But what I saw had shocked me completely.

His house was done up in the most vibrant, outrageous colours imaginable. His bedroom was painted a brilliant red. In the centre of it was a four-poster bed with a multi-hued bedspread. The Rajasthani mirror work on the canopy above the four-poster bed flashed colours of brilliant light everywhere. On the ornate bed were thrown several red pillows with a lot of brightly coloured tassels hanging from them.

His kitchen, surprisingly, was a bright pink. His flamboyant style floored me. But what really caught my attention was a picture. He had no photographs of any kind in his bedroom. Yet, mounted in a silver frame was a single picture—mine. I knew he was not only proud of me but also loved me deeply.

He had pooh-poohed the news of my cancer diagnosis and felt sure that I would be up on my feet stronger than before. His confidence made my heart sing.

Mama was a regular visitor during my treatment. One day, when he saw me feeling morose, confined to my bed, he promised to take me to a fashion show wearing his extravagant clothes. He said that my bald head would make a fashion statement.

I was undergoing chemotherapy at that time. Three rounds of my first session had been completed and my hair had started falling. While taking a shower, strands of hair would get stuck on the shower handle and taps and I would see clumps of it on my pillow when I woke up each morning. My mane was getting noticeably thinner. Yet it took me a while before deciding to go bald.

Finally, one day, I went to a salon and asked them to shave my hair off. I did not make a great deal of this decision. Of course it did pain me to see my hair gone, but I had made peace with myself on this issue. Zakia had explained to me that baldness would be a part of my treatment. So I was prepared for it. I had to tell myself that this was a small thing. I was more focused on making sure that the treatment was effective and on throwing the cancer cells out of my body. Mentally, I switched off from the pain and switched my mind on to the fact that if chemo was making me bald, it was also killing my cancer cells. I felt this was a small sacrifice to make.

That is why I smiled when Mama told me he would take me to a fashion show. I would wear one of his creations and my bald head would make a fashion statement. It thrilled me to be his muse. He had succeeded in tempting me. I eagerly looked forward to slipping my arm into the crook of his and enjoying the glamorous evening. I could not wait to get well. That is the kind of close bonding I had with him.

But that evening was never to be.

Months later, in February 2013, the news of his death reached me suddenly. My family had hidden it from me, and I accidentally stumbled on it. You can imagine my shock.

I sank into deep mourning. Shail Mama, though in his eighties, had the attitude and chutzpah of a youngster. How could a human dynamo like him die?

As if on cue, the clouds became dark and lightning flashed. I looked up at the New York sky.

Black clouds and white thunder. The black-and-white drama of nature appeared elemental. Was nature paying a tribute to that glorious human being? To the genius with a quirky sense of style?

The next instant, my mind rejected this tribute. What about the life he had led steeped in brilliant colours? Where had such a vibrant man disappeared?

I imagined him as a streak of merry breeze . . . a fast-moving meteor in the sky. I imagined him moving at a fast pace, diaphanous, stopping long enough to dip his brush into a huge tray of colours to paint the clouds an outrageous orange, pink and purple. Have you ever chanced on such clouds? Well, that's my beloved Mama's doing.

A sob rose from within me. New York would never be the same without him.

7

Surgery

10 December 2012

And, finally, it was the day of my surgery.

My mind kept playing the powerful, hope-filled exchange I had had with Dr Chi in a loop.

'Dr Chi, how long did that patient live?'

'She is alive and doing fine.'

I felt a rush of energy travelling through my veins, like swift little silverfish making their way upstream.

I had gone into the operation theatre riding on that wave of hope.

That morning at our hotel was tense. Nobody spoke. Yet we all understood. All of us headed towards the hospital quietly.

Reaching there at 10 a.m., we all felt that we had made the best choice. We also knew that we were yet to face the ordeal.

Within a few minutes of our arrival, I was wheeled into the holding area. My family stood by my side. We had to wait for around four hours before I would be taken into the anaesthesia room. It was an emotional moment for all of us. I could not find the right parting words to say.

Do not grieve too much for me?

or

I am so sorry I have put you all through so much pain.

or

Be strong. I'll be out and will be fine.

I said nothing. Instead, I looked lovingly at each person there in a bid to stamp their beloved faces on my heart.

I remember my friend Paulomi wrap her off-white shawl around me to keep me from shivering in the cold hospital room. I was touched by this gesture, for all of us knew that the shawl would be removed the moment I went inside and changed into the patient's uniform.

Without warning, the grim words that would be printed on Indian newspapers tomorrow flashed before my eyes: *Noted actor Manisha Koirala succumbs to cancer in New York.*

Horrified, I brushed that terrible thought away.

As I waited to be wheeled in, I thought to myself: *How bad would it actually be to die?*

Without warning, a funny thought emerged. Images of all those who had crossed over to the other side came to mind. They were actually giving me a champagne toast and telling me, 'You know, it's not too bad up here.'

All of them seemed bathed in golden sunlight and I could see right through them. I saw Karen Aunty smiling down at me. She was an Elizabeth Taylor lookalike and had a glass of champagne in her hand.

'It's not so bad this side, you know, Manisha!'

For a nanosecond, I actually wished I could join her there instead of being here in such pain and fear.

Soon, I was wheeled inside. The last thing I remember was seeing the kind, smiling face of nurse Nalini. She kept introducing herself and reassuring me in the sweetest way that everything would be fine. I slipped into a deep sleep.

Outside in the waiting room, my relatives paced anxiously. Dr Chi came out in his scrubs to speak with my mother and father.

Mom approached him nervously and very reluctantly asked him, 'I know you don't believe in this, but doctor, could you please keep this rudraksha mala with you while you perform the operation? We have faith that it can win over ill health.' She extended the mala towards him, afraid that he might refuse.

To further get her point across, she said, 'Lord Shiva will get you through the operation. Please help my daughter.'

Dr Chi smiled and nodded.

'I will keep it but I probably need to sterilize it first,' he said, smiling, and placed it in his pocket. 'You must worry only if I return quickly. If I take time, consider it a good sign,' he said reassuringly and turned to go.

Inside, in the sterile cold of the operation table, I faded in and out of anaesthesia, hallucinating that I was in a war zone. I was surrounded by tanks, artillery and fumes, the enemy flashing huge lights on me. *Why, I asked?* And then I slipped into unconsciousness.

The surgery lasted around eleven hours. Despite their worry and extreme exhaustion, my family kept their faith alive. They held on to the hope given by Dr Chi's words, 'Worry only if I return quickly.'

Outside, my mother kept chanting the powerful death-conquering mantra like one possessed:

Om tryambakam yajamahe sugandhim pustivardhanam . . .

She paced the floor, begging god to heal her precious daughter.

As the hours passed, exhausted, she fell asleep, chanting in the waiting room. A stranger tucked a pillow under her head and covered her with a blanket.

My father, an introvert, went out of the hospital into the snowy, windy night to talk to strangers. This was his way of dealing with his stress.

Thank god for caring relatives! Later on, Praveen Da, very methodically, captured the entire scene beautifully for me in an email I read later.

It was evening. We came down and sat in front of the waiting area facing the street. There, Nanu Di [my mom] crossed her legs on the sofa and began praying. She was dressed in heavy winter clothes. It was funny. The other visitors at the hospital hurriedly left that sofa area for us. Perhaps they thought we were Bin Laden followers—about to blow up the place.

Chetna went out with another relative, Mridula. I stayed behind with Nanu Di in case the doctor came looking for us. I had been through Chetna's surgeries several months ago and remembered the shock of the doctor coming out and telling me that she was critical. Thank goodness she had recovered and was with me tonight.

Later in the evening, we went to the upstairs waiting area and sat there until Dr Chi came. He told us we would get to visit you soon. But there was no one in the hospital and we went door to door looking for you. We finally found you in the recovery room at the back, towards the right-hand side. You were pretty much sedated.

When you came out of the recovery room to your hospital room in the morning, you looked very good. I remember the nurse telling us how beautiful you looked even after the surgery. I told her that you were once known as 'the prettiest face in Asia'. (P.S. So I don't get into trouble, you still are!) You gave us the thumbs up as I took the picture (which you have).

Overall, your dad remained very calm in the days before and during the surgery. In retrospect, however, I see that he must have been very troubled and was hiding his pain as he did not want to burden the family.

*That may have been why he kept going downstairs, outside in the cold, quite
often. It was snowing and the weather was harsh and windy. I could see
him going out to relieve his stress and talk to others. This was his way of
dealing with the turmoil.*

*Your bhai was managing everything and so he was able to keep his
mind on the logistics after your recovery. He probably bore the brunt of
everyone's frustration in the days following the surgery when things were
uncertain in terms of logistics, prep, etc. But as I told him then, he was
doing a great job overall and people were complaining to him as they were
all struggling to find a way to deal with your illness.*

It was almost 2 a.m. when Dr Chi came out of the theatre. My
anxious family huddled around him as if he were a war hero.

Quietly, he handed the rudraksha mala back to Mom and
said humbly, 'This mala has done the magic. The operation has
been successful.'

Praveen Da asked him, 'Will she recover?' To which Dr
Chi said, 'We have to be positive and assume full recovery.'

He explained to my family that the reason the surgery had
taken a long time was because the cancer had spread like a bowl
of Rice Krispies thrown all over the organs. He had to pick
them up one by one. He had performed an optimal debulking
surgery. He felt hopeful that 95 per cent—if not more—of the
cancer cells had been removed.

There was not a single dry eye surrounding Dr Chi at that
moment.

He informed my family that I would now be taken to the
recovery room and then to a hospital room the next morning
where the family would be able to meet me. But my mom insisted
that she wanted to see me right then, even if for a few minutes.

But it was twelve hours later that they finally got to see me—
through the glass window of the recovery room. Mom told me
later that she saw that my face was swollen and I was tethered

to an IV pole, monitors tracing the beats of my heart. She told me that when I sensed her near me, even in my unconscious state, I cried silent tears. Frantically, she made gestures at me. She kept signalling to me through the window to not cry. Her face was wet with tears, but she kept telling me that I would be fine.

That night, I was kept in the recovery room. I kept slipping in and out of consciousness. In one of my conscious moments, I recalled, with perfect clarity, the time I had met two Maori healers at a friend's apartment in Mumbai in June 2012. Those were the days when I used to be carefree.

In my friend's classy apartment, my mother and I had submitted our bodies to be examined by the two women healers. It just seemed such a cool, interesting thing to do. The main healer had checked my mom and immediately declared she was fine. The younger healer seemed puzzled when she began checking me. Her hands, hovering over my body, stopped just above my ovaries. Unsure, she checked again.

Then, she called the older Maori healer to be sure. The lady looked sombre after her hands hovered over me and said, 'Your ovaries are red hot. It seems like you are very angry with them. You need to send love to your ovaries.'

I had not taken her words seriously. I did not know how to send love to my ovaries. *Does anybody know that?* I simply shrugged and forgot about it.

But the import of that suddenly hit me now. The Maori healers had used their unique scanning system to diagnose me much before the doctors did!

Next morning, at 9.38 a.m., I was transferred to another room. I write this with precision because my uncle kept track of the exact time. That's what family members do.

I regained consciousness many hours later, but kept falling in and out of sleep. I was eager to talk to Dr Chi but he was nowhere to be seen.

Then, the following day, I finally woke up, fully conscious. I looked around and noticed that there were three beds in my room that could be divided into three separate sections by white curtains. There was a common bathroom for three patients.

I was lucky that I was on the far right. From my vantage point, I could see the sun filtering in through the window. In front of our beds was another window. I avoided looking at it. The only view was that of morose buildings. Above each bed there was a television. I did not want it switched on. I could sense multiple switches behind my bed. There were also gadgets to call the nurse or recline the bed myself.

I was confused and my eyelids felt heavy. My mouth just could not form the many questions I had. I looked up wearily.

I first saw Dad walk in. He was followed by the rest of my family. My eyes looked for my mother. Amidst the mayhem of my growing-up years and my tumultuous and hectic film career, she had been my solid rock. Today, I looked forward to receiving her brand of support and unconditional love. I needed them in huge doses today. I sought out her eyes. Her strong gaze has always been very reassuring for me.

My heart missed a beat.

She is going to tell me the good news. But why are her eyes averted? Why is she not smiling? Why is she not meeting my eyes with that happy, tender look she always gives me?

Where is Dr Chi—my saviour? What is happening?

Mom did not meet my eyes fully. I felt cold. But she smiled and the moment she took my hand into hers, I felt secure. The warmth of her fingers entwined into mine seemed to restore me to life.

An avid reader, I have always taken succour in literature, like a child running to its mother's lap. At that moment, Robert Frost's words from the poem 'Birches' seemed to speak to me about my state of swinging between life and death.

> And life is too much like a pathless wood
> Where your face burns and tickles with the cobwebs
> Broken across it, and one eye is weeping
> From a twig's having lashed across it open.
> I'd like to get away from earth awhile
> And then come back to it and begin over.

Dr Chi finally came to meet me on his rounds. I wanted to sit up, but found my body refusing to cooperate.

Perhaps now we will all laugh at it as if it were a bad dream. Perhaps now I will start living my life again.

But one look at him and I felt anxious. His face looked crestfallen; his eyes tired.

'What's wrong?' I asked, suddenly aware of the painful hollow in my stomach.

Quietly, holding my breath, I asked him, 'Was the surgery successful?'

There was total silence in the room. It was filled with my loved ones—my parents, some relatives, a few friends. But it was as if everybody were holding his or her breath. It was as if no one were in the room. We waited for Dr Chi's response.

'Yes,' he said quietly.

I smiled at Dr Chi and asked him brightly, 'So will I live for twenty-five more years?'

In my mind were stuck Zakia's hope-filled words. She had said to me that her cancer-afflicted sister was doing well even after twenty-five years. Dr Chi himself had mentioned that he knew a survivor who had lived that many years. I knew that he was always checking which of his patients had lived beyond twenty-five years. Thus it became a standard in my head.

He shrugged his shoulders. Silence again.

'Then?'

'During the surgery, I saw the extent of how much your cancer had spread. I wasn't expecting it. We took out everything we could. So in that sense the surgery was successful. But I don't know how well you will react to chemo, so I can't say,' he explained. 'Cancer is not like cough and cold—I can't tell you for certain if taking some medication will cure it completely. I need to know how well you will respond to the chemo for me to honestly answer that question,' he explained.

His words made my heart sink.

This very doctor had given me hope. How unfair that now I had to wait for chemotherapy to find out whether I had a chance at life?

I had felt so hopeful just a few minutes ago. And here was my doctor telling me it wasn't going to be. I looked around at everyone, and that's when I realized that my loved ones had known it all along. While I was surfacing from and sinking into my anaesthetic sleep, they had been told.

I felt tears welling up inside me. Emotions clamoured to express themselves, fighting past the operated emptiness of my mutilated body.

Was I going to live? Was I going to die? This state of not knowing was the worst.

8

Dr Makker Enters My Life

'Life is filled with detours and dead-ends, trials and challenges of every kind. Each of us has likely had times when distress, anguish, and despair almost consumed us.'

—Russell M. Nelson

Have you ever wondered what emotions a cancer patient goes through? Let me tell you that they are probably worse than what a prisoner on death row feels.

Of course there is a feeling of gloom and doom. But there is also the feeling of extreme hopelessness, helplessness and powerlessness.

Your physical body—the one you either took for granted or took pride in as your ally suddenly betrays you, leaving you shocked.

Your mind, which wove dreams and plans for your future, unexpectedly finds that everything has come to a standstill.

And your spirit? Not too long back it soared. It now lies defeated and punctured, trapped within your physical boundaries, enslaved to a bed.

Yet, very much like a prisoner on death row, a strange flicker of hope continues to burn timidly in the wounded heart. Like the feeble wick of an oil lamp fighting against a strong breeze. Both the prisoner and the patient hope desperately for a reprieve—a magical intervention from a higher force which, at the last moment, will save them from death.

In my case, I felt that magical person was going to be Dr Vicky Makker, who Dr Chi had referred me to.

On the morning following my operation, my body felt strange. It was a mass of conflicting sensations. I was on pins and needles. At once light and heavy, weak and strong, familiar and unfamiliar, identifiable and nameless, mine and not mine. I could move my fingers. Also my toes. Yet the length of my body felt broken and repaired, fragmented and smashed, disjointed and jerky. And, despite the painkillers, that heavy, numbing pain remained a constant. My mouth tasted acrid. Dr Chi's words had sent my spirits dashing to the ground. My last hope was this new doctor. There were two things in her favour: first, she was a woman, and second, she was a young Punjabi of Indian origin. I felt that my comfort level with a woman doctor of Indian origin would be more. Not that her being a woman mattered to me much, but her being of Indian origin did make me feel relieved. She would probably have heard of me. This would make it easier for me to ask questions. I could confide in her about my worries. I hoped we could be friends. In fact I felt certain she would become not only my soul-sister but also my saviour, my redeemer, my life-giver.

Dr Makker had received her medical degree from the University of Florida College of Medicine and had been practising for almost twenty years. I felt fortunate that I would be under her experienced care at the hospital.

She had received great reviews on Vitals.com. The comments under 'Patient Reviews' said she was 'amazing', 'very knowledgeable', 'caring' and 'professional'. Now that suited me just fine. I was ready to become her best friend for life.

Those were my emotions when this stunning woman, garlanded with a stethoscope, walked in. She looked confident, on top of her game, and smiled brightly. Not a hair was out of place, neither was a single tooth in that dazzling even row of white. What really caught my attention, however, were the strikingly huge solitaire diamonds she wore on her ears.

For a minute, I could not help the fashionista in me from surfacing. I too love diamonds. I have noticed that most Indians love rock diamonds, unlike Westerners. I have always joked about the fact that a small house could be bought from the shine on our earlobes.

So that means our tastes are similar. Another reason why we will bond!

In a bid to charm her and acknowledge our mutual fashion sense, I pointed to her ears and said, 'Those are pretty. I love them!'

She flashed a bright smile back and said, 'I love the man who gave them to me!'

Having established our mutual ground, I quickly figured our relationship out in my head. This angel would take care of me tenderly. She would comfort me, bond with me and hold my hand lovingly through several rounds of chemotherapy. I kept smiling in a knowing manner, all the time looking at her. But what my eyes saw did not match the image in my head.

What's wrong? Why is she not responding with the same warmth? Why is she going out of her way to be distant, aloof, strict? Why is she not behaving like my soul-sister?

I was dismayed that she simply did not see me as her BFF! I asked her in a back-to-business voice to give me statistics about the survival rates for late-stage ovarian cancer patients.

She looked directly into my eyes and did not mince any words: 'The statistics are not good, Manisha. The five-year survival rate is . . .' My mind froze the moment she said five.

What she said after that got lost in the flood that arose within me. I could see her speaking, moving her lips. But the content eluded me completely.

I interpreted that she meant I would live up to five years at best. I burst into tears.

I was not even going to live five years?

I could see my mom stepping forward to hold me and console me.

'Beta, that is not what she meant . . .'

But I did not care for any explanations. Nothing registered in my brain. I was done with receiving bad news all the time. It had come pouring in at me: first the doctor in Kathmandu, then Dr Advani in Mumbai and then Dr Chi in New York.

My last hope had been Dr Makker. She too had shattered my fragile hold on optimism. I wanted to scream, to run away, to do something outrageous.

My emotions were in shreds. They had been on a rollercoaster ride for far too long. It's not easy to live constantly under the shadow of looming death.

As a child, I remember once watching a magnificent, gloriously coloured butterfly perch blissfully on a flower. Its beautiful blue wings reminded me of the stained glass windows of a church. Daintily, it sucked nectar from the red flower, as if from a straw, its wings folded neatly upwards.

Just then, before my horrified eyes, a noisy group of girls broke into the idyllic scene. They captured this unsuspecting 'flower in the sky' and swiftly, stuffed it into a glass jar with a very tiny hole.

'Caught another one!' they giggled triumphantly, ignoring my protests.

I looked sadly at the butterfly flapping its brilliant coloured wings inside the glass jar. Born to fly freely in the sky, it felt puzzled by the imprisonment. It began struggling furiously to escape. With its fragile, delicate, flimsy wings flapping, it flew to the top of the jar, willing it to open . . . again and again.

The brave butterfly, despite its air supply getting cut off, kept trying. I noticed how its wings looked like painted silk and as delicate as rice paper. It was born beautiful, but now destined to die.

My heart went out to it. I could empathize with its struggle for survival . . . Its struggle to breathe . . . its struggle to be free. I could relate perfectly with its agony.

I too felt exactly like it. Trapped. With no hope of escape.

9

How Bollywood Came to My Rescue

'Everyone wants attention, more or less. I just want a lot.'
—*Zara Larsson*

I imagined a black-robed, white-haired judge sitting above, awarding me life in ten-day blocks. First there had been a ten-day wait before my operation. Now there was going to be a ten-day wait at the hospital while I recovered. Perhaps there would be another ten-day gap before I could start the dreaded chemotherapy sessions.

So here I was, lying on my hospital bed, feeling completely dependent on the nurses for my movement. I was anxious and in pain—not only physically, emotionally too. Not knowing what lay ahead, I surrendered to going with the flow. I began taking each moment as it came. Swinging between life and death, I had plenty of time to be alone with my thoughts. My mind went back to the charmed life I had led in Mumbai.

I entered the world of films in 1991 with the top-grossing *Saudagar*, a dream break by any standards. With a mentor of the stature of Subhash-ji, life could not have been more perfect. The audience immediately sat up and noticed the new Nepalese girl and many sang praises of her innocent beauty.

Money, name, fame and a string of hits—I had it all. I had friends whom I could party with at any time and awards that were coveted by many. It was a life only the chosen few get to live.

But even though the world was at my feet, something strange began happening to me. I soon started feeling the misery of existence. I became wretched.

I think it was during the shooting of *Laawaris*, which released in 1999, that I felt the pressure getting to me. I had been working non-stop till then. I confided in Dimple Kapadia that I was tired of this routine of getting up, putting on make-up, going out for location shooting, returning home exhausted and being constantly 'on the go'.

Without my realizing it, my life went into a downward spiral. I quickly lost interest in the privileges that were being bestowed on me. I became bored and disinterested in life. The pressure of performing so many roles, of expressing so many emotions every single day, began to vex me. I became a robot—instantly donning another persona at the snap of 'Lights, Camera, Action'.

I became tired of the relentless pattern of my days—wake up, shower, put on make-up, work, come home, remove make-up, sleep. I think I felt the final snap at the point I was acting in twelve films in a year. The pressure was too much. The burden began seeping into my bones; the complexities of my characters began gnawing at my soul. There was no holiday, no time to watch the clear blue skies and golden beaches. Just constant trips to the film set and the hotel.

I remember how resentful I had felt when I had gone for a shoot in Australia. I wanted to immerse myself in the timelessness of the Great Barrier Reef, the MacKenzie Falls, the Kakadu National Park and the stunning landscapes.

I wished to run outdoors to explore the bushwalking trails and soak in the beauty of the Blue Mountains. For I hail from the mountains myself and have been an ardent nature lover all my life.

Instead, I was shepherded out of Mumbai, taken to the film set, asked to memorize my lines and perform and promptly flown out of the country to yet another film set.

Was I enjoying getting up at unearthly hours? Was I ecstatic about visiting so many countries? Was I appreciative of all these opportunities? No. I felt like an automaton, reduced to being a pretty face. I think that's when my mind began to get toxic. Emotionally, I began to go into reverse.

To take my mind off shoots, to numb myself, I started drinking. If I was on a diet, it would be vodka. I remember my ex-boyfriend once telling me that I had no sense of balance. He said, 'You are a workaholic. You either work hard or party hard. Where is your sense of balance?'

Of course I was aware that I had a tendency to go overboard. Many people around me had tried to tell me that.

But the truth is that I wasn't enjoying it. I didn't appreciate my work. I simply didn't like it. Somewhere, in a contorted way, I began wilfully doing the wrong things. To spite myself, I chose the wrong films. I began feeding my ego.

I insisted on being the central character, even if it was in a B-grade film. At that point, I did not even care who the director was. Getting a central role mattered more than anything else.

My state of mind was toxic, my approach to life complacent and my attitude ungrateful. So here I was, reliving the past in my head in a hospital in New York, praying desperately that I would live.

I snapped out of my reverie abruptly when one of the nurses came up to me and asked me to stand up.

What? How does she even imagine I can do that? Everything hurts so badly. I just can't! And won't!

Of course I understood that the nurses wanted me to move my body to begin the healing process. They encourage you to either walk in the hospital corridor or move around a bit to begin the curative and restorative effects post-surgery.

The next moment my hard taskmaster made me do exactly what she had in mind. I clenched my teeth at the onrush of pain. I all but collapsed. Then stand I did, on legs that seemed to be made of jelly. The torture did not end there. On the third day, a nurse came up to me early in the morning and said, 'Come on, honey, let's walk to the washroom and take a shower.'

I was horrified. I protested. She was adamant.

She handed me a walker and insisted I ignore the pain.

'Oh, it's not too bad, honey!'

I summoned up all my courage. Using superhuman effort, I put one foot in front of the other. The pain made me grimace. But the nurse was calm—in a strict, no-nonsense manner. She expected me to walk towards the bathroom as casually as if I were taking a morning stroll.

Once there, she got busy taking my hospital robe off.

I let out a raspy, guttural scream the moment I saw my naked body reflected in the bathroom mirror. What had happened to my marble-white satin skin? My flesh had been ruthlessly stapled with steel pins right from below my breasts to my groin.

Is this really my body?

My head spun, my knees gave way and I collapsed.

Very professionally, the nurse steadied me and gently led me forward until I was seated on the toilet seat, groaning with the effort of so much movement. And the shock of seeing my maimed body.

'There, there!' she said and clucked like a mother goose. I tried to collect myself. But my body would not cooperate.

Ignoring my discomfort, she began to bathe me expertly with the help of a hand shower. Professionally, she manoeuvred through the jagged route of the horrific steel staples that kept my body from splitting apart.

I was overcome by weakness—physical, emotional, mental. I felt really sorry for myself. However, that left no impression on the caring nurses. They made me go through this routine every single day.

One day, however, overcome by emotion and weakness, I slipped in the bathroom. The attending nurse rushed to help me and called out to the other nurses to give her a hand. Together, they carried me back to my bed.

I realized then that I was just a mass of flesh and blood—mutilated and broken inside out. More than doctors, I was now completely dependent on nurses to make me whole again. The realization was a humbling one.

One night I needed a nurse urgently. I rang the bell several times to call the nurse on duty. I was anxious and the wait seemed endless.

This is no good. I need to think of a ploy.

To tell you the truth, with each passing day, I was becoming stronger. That is why my mind was clear enough to implement a strategy, and Bollywood came to my rescue.

The next day, when the morning-shift nurse arrived, I began making small talk with her—the light and breezy kind that connects one woman to another.

Shamelessly, I resorted to name-dropping. Mine!

'Have you heard of India's Bollywood?' I asked the nurse as she pulled out and reapplied my wound dressing quite mechanically.

'You mean in which they dance and sing? Ah, yes! I love watching those musicals.'

'Well, I am a big star there, you know. I have done eighty films in Bollywood.'

She paused, mid-action. I could see a veil of admiration descending on her bored eyes. She looked at me with new eyes now.

She checked my vitals more attentively, smiled at me more and even placed the TV remote in my hands!

My heart rejoiced as I stroked the length and breadth of the TV remote. It had worked!

After that, I began dropping gems of information about my starry life on my attending nurses. The result? I would receive more sympathy and extra care from them. I could even ask for and become the privileged recipient of more heated blankets whenever I fancied them.

'Really?' the nurses would ask me. I would nod my head, trying to look important and yet being very matter-of-fact about it.

My clever plan had worked, but it drained my energy. I had to use the same strategy shift after shift.

'Why don't you Google me?' I asked them, hoping they would give me more attention.

My fairy-tale introduction actually worked as an open sesame. They suddenly became curious about me and the enchanted life I had led. It opened the door to many deep conversations, surprisingly. We shared our joys, sorrows, concerns, fears and hopes and spoke about the situations we currently found ourselves in.

From a patient–nurse relationship, we graduated into one of woman to woman. I got into a first-name basis with each of them. We joked, laughed, prayed and kept track of what was going on in each other's lives on a day-to-day basis. We discovered each other's human side. The bonds between us became personal.

My head clearer now, I began noticing the flowers that would arrive in my room and told them stories about the people who had sent them. As I began to feel better, I also noticed the cards from fans, family and friends that arrived in the mail for me. The nurses would carefully prop them all up in neat arrangements in my room.

Grateful and delighted at this attention, I would say loudly to them: 'Are they all beautiful? Any particular one stands out?' It was a game we played happily each morning and afternoon.

With my new-found friendship, the days began to fly quickly. One by one, the tubes connected to my body began to be removed, much to my relief. There was only one prominent one inserted into my lungs for draining excess fluid. That took a long time to go.

But eventually, one day, there remained no more appendages and tentacles attached to me. The wounds that still looked frightening to me were now bandaged up tightly, waiting to be taken off after the healing was complete.

One day, another renowned doctor came visiting me— Dr Navneet Narula, fondly known as Zeena-ji. She was a pathologist at Cornell Medical Centre. Dr Narula was unpretentious and straightforward. Methodically, she went through every report—the doctors' as well as the lab's.

All the time, I kept my eyes focused on her face to gauge her reaction.

Suddenly, her eyes filled with tears and she looked away from me. I saw her wipe her tears. My heart sank.

Later, I heard that she mentioned to her husband, Dr Jagat Narula, how grave my medical reports were. Also, her admiration for how composed and calm I was despite knowing that.

Nothing in my life has gone smoothly.

One day I was informed that the ghastly staples would be removed from my body. Post-surgery, the doctors had stapled my skin after stitching it to keep it together while it healed—much like stapled paper. My entire torso had been opened and from the stomach down, I was stapled up. When I got to know that these were going to be removed, I became a bundle of nerves. My heartbeats became mad and irregular, my palms sweaty and there was that old sinking feeling.

No more pain, god. Please. No more pain!

A tiny sigh of relief escaped my lips when I saw the nurse who had come to do the job. I liked her and knew all about her life. She smiled at me reassuringly and I relaxed. She had earlier given me an injection and had done it so painlessly that I had admired her expertise. I was happy that she would be removing my staples. I was certain she would be kind to me. At least I prayed she would.

As always, I began to hide my nervousness by blabbering away. I assumed that our chit-chats would make her more sympathetic and kind towards me.

Flippantly, I popped several everyday questions at her. I acted normal and friendly, as if cutting off steel staples from my tender flesh was a daily game I enjoyed playing.

In a bright, high-pitched voice that belied my trembling body, I asked casually, 'So, what did you have for lunch?'

We could well have been sitting in my house, exchanging pleasantries over green tea.

I did not know if she was listening. I did not even know if I expected to find out the answer to my world-shaking query. She was focused on only the task at hand.

Suddenly I felt a painful snip on my stomach.

Wincing in pain, I asked once again, 'So how are your kids?'

Again another snip.

I gritted my teeth.

'And your work?'

Snip, she went again, until I realized what a silly question that was. *This* was her work. And this was what she was doing right then. But I kept asking random questions. Anything to take my mind off from the pain.

Each time she snipped with her steel pincers, I yelped loudly. She had not spoken until then. But now she did. She stopped mid-snip, looked me straight in the eye—her blue ones locking with my brown ones—and asked, 'Is it really hurting? Or are you just scared?'

I paused, feeling like a child who had been caught and reprimanded. I took a deep breath.

Am I just afraid or am I in pain?

The discovery made me snap my eyes open. A frisson of shame rushed through me. Yes, there was no pain, just fear.

So I resolved to become more mature. As she went about the process of de-stapling me, I trained my mind to not listen to the clipping sound any more. I clenched my jaws. Wilfully, I diverted my mind to other worries—bigger ones. God knows I had enough of them.

After a long session of gritting my teeth silently and scraping my palms with my nails, the ordeal was finally over. All the staples had been removed.

But when I looked down at my bruised body, I was shocked.

In the centre of my body were two gaping holes—crater-like, cavernous depressions. Horrified and traumatized, I looked at the nurse in confusion, my swollen lips unable to form the right words.

She replied nonchalantly, as if we were witnessing a piece of art, 'You shouldn't be scared of these; what is inside you is far more dangerous.'

Her last sentence left me gulping for air.

* * *

Finally, it was time to leave the hospital. There were a zillion papers to be signed. I could see my brother running around trying to complete the formalities.

As for myself, I felt strange. I lay in bed and looked at the hospital room that had been my home for so long. I thought of the kind faces of the nurses who had so charmingly switched over from being mere caregivers to caring friends.

I felt a twinge of regret at leaving everything I had become accustomed to.

I remember shaking myself. Was I experiencing something like the Stockholm Syndrome—a psychological condition in which the prisoner becomes overly fond of its captors and does not want to leave them? I had read a story about a hostage who developed a psychological bond with his captors as a survival strategy during captivity. It was scary, if not funny.

Paperwork over, I was overcome with gratitude and relief. As I was wheeled out, I noticed that the big lobby of the hospital was filled with smiling nurses. Regardless of what the future had in store for me, I felt happy at that moment. The worst was over (my operation). So what if the worst (chemotherapy) remained? It was still ten days away.

The chemotherapy session would take place in a different wing of the hospital. I would not meet these nurses there.

I went over to each sister and hugged them warmly. I presented each of them with colourful flowers (our talking points!) that had spread happiness and fragrance in my room. I was grateful for the cheer they had brought me.

Joy radiated from each of us and wrapped us closely in a strong bond. I told each one of them how lucky I was to have had such amazing caregivers and how saying goodbye to them seemed so hard.

A change had begun taking shape within me during my stay at the hospital. I started becoming more appreciative of each moment. I learnt the art of picking up each moment carefully, diving inside it, admiring its possibilities and experiencing it fully before stringing it back with the other pearls on the necklace of time. I realized I had become a moment-to-moment person, filled with a deep appreciation for every little bit that life generously handed to me.

Gently, I told myself the words I had heard somewhere: Today I open the door to the future, take a deep breath, step on through and start a new chapter in my life.

10

New Apartment Joys

'Hope smiles from the threshold of the year to come, whispering, "It will be happier."'

—*Alfred Lord Tennyson*

'Lots of air, sunshine and no dark corners' were the list of criteria I had given Bhai when he started looking for an apartment for us to stay in after leaving the Plaza. I was just giving voice to my soul.

After listing it out, my lips curled into a smile. My baby brother had evolved into a responsible young man during this entire crisis. Earlier, I liked to think that I was his protector. Suddenly, there had been a role reversal.

In his growing-up years, I had almost been a mother figure to him. When Mom and Dad were away from Nepal for some time, he had come over to stay with me in Mumbai. During this period, I became his mom, teacher, guide and friend. Our relationship remained like that. In any crisis, he would look up to his *didi* and I would be there for him.

Yet now his beloved sister was flat on her back, incapable of taking any decisions. My parents were equally nervous and shaken up. Bhai realized that he had to now lead the family out of this crisis. So he took on the reins in his hands—running around to fill out the countless forms required for admitting international patients, completing all the paperwork, handling our finances, paying bills, arranging cars, setting up appointments with doctors and nurses, checking the medicines and doing everything that needed to be done. He took complete control of the situation.

Since he was the youngest in the group, he was at the receiving end of everyone's complaints and demands. Everyone wanted something to be organized, something to be done. His own sister had certain requirements for the apartment's location, appeal and aesthetics. He had to run around in an unfamiliar city to find the right place. I can imagine the pressure on his young shoulders. He also had to take a lot of flak, like anyone who has to do so much and cater to so many people is bound to get. But he never once complained, nor lost his calm. He felt hugely responsible.

My eyes fill up with tears even now when I recall those days. I am overcome with admiration for my brattish young brother who emerged as a mature, responsible man in the face of a family crisis. For the first time I saw my little brother transform into a level-headed man. He truly rose to the occasion and I feel so very proud of him.

It had been planned that after my operation and subsequent discharge from the hospital, we would shift to an apartment in a week. We had taken this decision because my immune system was going to get weaker after chemotherapy. Sanitization would become crucial. Mom would also be able to cook food for me in an apartment of our own.

Of course, I was nervous about moving out because of the comfort the hotel provided. Help was just a call away. In the interest of my likely weakness and compromised immune system, however, we had to take the decision to move out.

We wanted to be closer to the hospital in case any emergency occurred. I had a few relatives in Jackson Heights and New Jersey and they had graciously offered their homes to me. But I knew we needed a place near the hospital. Apartment prices, however, are steep around Manhattan.

So there were two battles ahead: first was moving homes and the second was chemo. But in my newly discovered resolve to become a 'moment-to moment' person, I decided to make the most of my week at the Plaza.

Mom could not bear to look at the hideous wounds on my stomach, and I still felt dizzy when I did. So we had to find a home-care specialist who would come to dress my wounds. And thus we found Sheila, a residential nurse. She was efficient and made me feel comfortable.

But the stitches did not hold my stomach well.

'Why are the holes still there?' I asked her.

'It's probably some stitching inside gone awry. But don't you worry, these are all soluble stitches and they will heal soon.'

I realized I would just have to wait it out.

Intezaar is a Hindi word that I feel describes perfectly the endless spells of waiting a cancer patient has to go through. Usually a confident, impatient person who likes to get things done fast, I had been subjected to large doses of it. I had gone through it in Kathmandu, waiting for Dr Ghimire's report; I had experienced it during my nail-biting wait for Dr Advani's, Dr Chi's and Dr Makker's opinions about the gravity of my condition; and I now had to wait for these gaping holes on my body to heal before I could start my last shot at life— chemotherapy. Okay, I sighed. I would endure the healing of my wounds too.

In its wisdom, time was gently replacing my impulsiveness with maturity; the old controlling-me with the new surrendering-me. I was surprised how I was actually going with the flow.

This time too Sahara Shree's people, among others, came to my rescue, helping us move into a comfortable apartment near the hospital's emergency section. My brother had worked very hard to find the right flat.

So finally we bade goodbye to the luxury of Plaza Hotel and moved into our new apartment. It was a small two-bedroom flat with balconies, a living room and an open kitchen. The entire building had a positive vibe. It even had a small park attached to it, which my brother felt suited me fine if I could not go on long walks.

It was late December by the time we moved—Dad, Mom, my brother and I. I was looking forward to ringing in the New Year here with my family.

My body was still weak. But my mind told me that I must prepare it for the long battle ahead. New York lay glittering in the afterglow of Christmas and the anticipation of New Year.

* * *

I have always been 'Daddy's girl' since childhood. I can only imagine the pain he went through on seeing me in that condition. But not once did he put it into words. Even now, if I ask him about it, he will probably not make a big deal of it. He has never been one to complain or express his feelings if he is in any kind of discomfort. That is why none of us can ever know what he is actually going through unless one is very observant. But my uncle and brother can vouch for the way he handled his own grief so silently and in such a dignified manner.

Dad has been a voracious reader and is a very well-read man. During those days, he would read one newspaper several times over. That was his only way of coping. If the day's newspaper did not come in, he would continue reading the old one over and over. Or whatever he could lay his hands on. He did not know how else to handle his sorrow.

The anxiety of possibly losing his precious daughter had made a big difference to his daily routine. He could not bring upon himself to step out to get the newspaper. He drowned his sorrow in reading the old ones again and again. This silent activity became his refuge. When later my brother told me this, it hit me hard.

Before my illness, he would sip some wine once in a while but he stopped that habit completely. Slowly, once the initial shock had seeped in, he began going out for early morning walks. On one of these outings, he discovered a Bangladeshi newspaper stall nearby. Gradually, he included evening walks into his routine too.

But Dad took time to get used to this routine. Back from his walk, he would come back quietly and sit with me. Most of the time, however, he would be in his own space, slightly away from me, yet keeping an eye on me.

Dad became our inspiration for leading a healthy lifestyle. He still is an epitome of good health and we love him more for it.

* * *

A few days after moving into our own space, I peeped outside. A snowstorm was building up and made everything look pretty. With a jolt, I realized that I had not stepped out of the apartment in a long time.

What a pity, I thought! When it was sunny, I had been unwell and now when my strength was coming back, it had begun to snow!

So I decided on two things. First, I would walk either in my corridor or in my room for at least thirty minutes a day. I had spent the previous day just watching TV. This was not helping me. Staying in my bed, I felt weak and miserable. I felt alone.

Second, I would work on my posture. After surgery, I had begun to stoop a little. This was not good at all. I did not want to form a lifelong habit of stooping. So I decided to correct my posture and get rid of my stoop.

* * *

For me, family time is always celebration time. With New Year round the corner and a person as effervescent as Shail Mama to keep us in high spirits, we were in a festive mood. To add to the cheer, Mama brought along a gift for everyone—designer caps, mufflers, gloves, socks and ties. We had a merry time trying each one out. There was a lot of laughter.

Finally, it was midnight. The old year was gone. A new year had dawned. Not any day, but a New Year's Day. As everyone around me hugged and wished each other, I became pensive.

Life was offering me a fresh new start. A new chapter was waiting to be written. On my life's freshly opened page, I decided *I* was going to be the writer. It would be a transformative year for me, one in which I would take the controls back into my hands. It would be a year of embracing, forgiving and loving.

I would ask new questions and hug new answers, however frightening they might appear to be. I would delight in my self-discovery. I would dream once more.

That's when I stated my brave New Year resolution: *I will live.*

11

Chemotherapy

'Waiting is painful. Forgetting is painful. But not knowing which to do is the worst kind of suffering.'

—*Paulo Coelho*

After my operation, much before my chemo started, Dr Makker invited me to her chamber to check my wound. The two holes on my stomach had not yet healed after the operation and needed to be dressed every day by a nurse. Through it, I could see something white inside. I did not know whether it was pus or something else.

Dr Makker explained the process of chemotherapy. I was informed that in the next six months, I would be given eighteen sessions of chemo. I trembled.

After that, a nurse gave me a paper to sign. My horrified eyes read the dangers I was exposing myself to by agreeing to get chemotherapy done. Permanent heart damage, permanent ear damage, permanent neuropathic problems, blackening of the nails, a metallic taste in the mouth and the possibility of shaky hands throughout my life.

'Then why?' I asked mournfully to the nurse who had given me the paper.

'So that we can hope your cancer does not come back,' she explained.

That silenced me.

I desperately tried to un-learn whatever I had read. But the horrible images of what I could turn into kept whirring in my brain, like a swarm of angry bees.

Despite how I felt, I was in a hurry to begin my chemotherapy sessions. A twinge of disappointment pricked at me when I learnt that my first chemo appointment, scheduled for 2 January, had been postponed because my freshly operated body was weak and still under attack. The two gaping holes in my abdomen hadn't healed. Chemo at that time would have not only delayed the healing process but also put me at risk of contracting some infection.

Finally, on 8 January, my doctor decided to go ahead with my session in spite of my open wounds. I remember her saying that any delay could be fatal.

The thought of putting chemical substances into my body made me turn icy cold. I do not know how people can remain brave through this process. I was not.

I felt as if I were falling into a bottomless void—like free matter drifting in space.

I recalled the feelings I had gone through earlier while waiting for my blood work (the American term for blood tests). Compared to the general section, the women's section, where I would wait for my tests or appointments, was fairly empty.

I remember noticing that on one side were the cancer patients—grim and sombre-looking with specks of death floating in their weary eyes. On the other were the nurses—smiling gloriously and bursting forth with life. I remember noticing their high fashion boots and sparkling eyes.

I felt an invisible line dividing us—the world of dying patients and the world of the living.

When had I crossed that invisible line?

* * *

As a family, on the day before my chemo, we fell silent. Words became redundant. Only feelings lay heavy, like a quilt, suffocating us with its weight.

The day we had all been dreading, 8 January, finally dawned. I watched Mom prepare a healthy breakfast for us all. She woke up at 4 a.m. to bathe and pray for mercy to the divine. The house smelt of incense sticks—I think it was *mogra* (jasmine) that tickled us with its smell. Quickly, she checked to see if I had dressed appropriately. I had. I wore a loose dress—since I had been told by the doctors that my stomach would bloat—a cap and a borrowed winter coat.

Our family friend Biru had flown in from Delhi to accompany us to the hospital. Bhai had arranged cabs for all of us. Hurriedly, we got into them and Bhai asked the drivers to take us to 53rd Street between Third and Lexington.

New York scenes whizzed past me. I was completely wrapped up in my cocoon of fear. On reaching the hospital, we stopped at a different section of Sloane. This was the chemo centre. I was in a complete daze—like a lamb being taken to a slaughterhouse. All I wanted was to curl up and die.

When we walked into the chemo centre I was sure we all looked quite a sight—eight sad-looking Asians walking solemnly, their lips moving in soundless prayer.

We were met by Dr Makker. She looked amused, yet stern.

'Manisha, you need to have fewer people around you. There is space for only two in the chemo area.'

As if on cue, all others faded guiltily into the background as Mom accompanied me in.

My respect for Mom went up by leaps and bounds during this period. As a child, living with my grandmother, I had never discovered this side of her. But now I was amazed by her unwavering focus on my welfare. Her determination was strong. As were her prayers. I trusted her to be my intermediary with the divine, putting forth strong arguments of why I should be spared.

I lay quietly in my room, lost in my thoughts, clinging to the security I drew from my *tulsi bead mala*. Everything around me seemed to be collapsing. Only the touch of the hard, grainy beads was reassuring. I had been told that the 108 beads on the mala represented the different stages of the human soul's journey, each being progressive and on a continuum. There is often an overlap between each of these phases— *sariyai, kiriyai, yogam* and *jnanam*—until one finally merges with god. The 108 beads are strung along with a 'guru bead', the beads turning like planets around the sun as the mantra is repeated.

In Hinduism, the number 108 has profound significance. It is considered the number of the wholeness of existence. The average distance of the sun and moon to earth is 108 times their respective diameters; there are 108 *pithas*, or sacred sites, throughout India in yogic tradition; 108 Upanishads; 108 *marma* points, or sacred places, in the body; and 108 sun salutations can be offered in a yoga mala.

O divine, if this is the final stage of my journey in this physical life, I beg you to make it painless. I have suffered enough for one lifetime.

Sweat poured down my cheeks. I wiped it off with fingers that were ice-cold.

Will my body be able to withstand this onslaught? And for how long?

* * *

At first it was just one vicious wolf hurtling forward at top speed inside me.

And suddenly there was a pack of them. Dark, wild wolves, their mouths open, fangs bared, seeking out each vein of my body, tearing forward at great speed, hell-bent on destruction.

Hungrily, they began devouring everything in sight—my organs, my blood, my veins, my bones. It was maddening. I knew I would not live through this. My face became flushed, my skin broke out in angry rashes. My stomach hurt and I had a strong desire to throw up.

The nurses panicked.

'The blood pressure is up—the heart rate is shooting up! Stop the infusion!'

An authoritative voice called out: 'Page Dr Makker urgently! Get her here! Tell her it's an emergency!'

* * *

As I lay in the hospital bed, I trembled. I had two ports inserted into my body to infuse the drugs—one was below my right shoulder and the other on my left side, near my stomach. The nurse on duty came and put a tube into one of the ports. I shut my eyes.

O merciful divine! Let the process be painless please!

I heard my mom's chants floating into the room. I felt drugged. I think I even drifted into a fitful sleep.

At some point, the heavy chemotherapy liquid began dripping into my body.

And then, its horrible reactions.

I felt intense heat coming out of my stomach. It began to hurt badly. My body burst into red rashes. My heart began to pound. I was overcome by sudden nausea and lower back pain.

I knew I was having an allergic reaction.

'Call Dr Makker! Quick!'

When Dr Makker arrived a few minutes later, she seemed visibly upset with the developments. She had not expected my body to react in this manner to the drugs.

Heart pounding, breathing ragged, vision blurred, I lay quietly—a mask of calmness on my face.

Seeing her visibly shaken, I mustered up courage and spoke in a voice trembling with pain, 'Doc, can you please change the chemo? Obviously this concoction is not working.'

I had read on the Internet that some people react very badly to chemotherapy. Some patients have allergic reactions and in such cases the body rejects the medicines. I do not remember where exactly I had read this as I had become a compulsive googler and kept reading a lot about my condition and treatment. As you know, when you are driven by fear, your eyes seek out only negative things on the Net.

Dr Makker looked amused, but stern: 'This cocktail of drugs is the best for your kind of cancer. Let me do what I know best. I am going to give it another try. You should be fine.'

I was beyond caring. My body was now feeling numb. I remember being given a medicine to make me drowsy.

I looked at Dr Makker through the haze of drowsiness, like a defeated prisoner.

I was surprised to see how confident and gritty she was. With great earnestness she said, 'Manisha, please do not worry.

I am 100 per cent with you. This mix is right for you—it is the best choice for your cancer type.' With her sitting there, I felt slightly more confident.

An hour later, she infused Benadryle into me to calm my nerves. Then she administered the same chemotherapy cocktail very slowly—drop by drop. She had explained to me earlier that this was a 'first-priority drug' for my condition. Thankfully, my body did not go into shock this time and I had no allergic reaction. The session went off smoothly. In fact I became so relaxed that I slept off. Dr Makker remained constantly by my side.

Around five hours later, we drove back to our apartment.

Surprisingly, my head was filled with thoughts of not my allergic reaction to the infusion but of Dr Makker. I had seen her in a new light that day and I liked what I saw. She possessed a razor-sharp mind and knew exactly how to handle emergencies.

My first chemo session had made my confidence in myself dip. I had pretended to be confident while actually I was gripped by fear. The allergic reaction had shaken me up.

Yet, after seeing how expertly Dr Makker had handled the crisis—insisting that I take the same drug under her supervision—I felt relieved. My doctors knew exactly what to do with me. That raised my confidence in them.

With these professionals, I felt safe.

* * *

With no option left, I decided to become a 'professional patient'. Diligently, I began obeying every instruction given to me. I told myself several times that each session was meant to destroy my errant cells permanently. That gave me hope.

But the feeling of pessimism and despair refused to leave me. It was gloomy and cold outside. So was my mood.

I desperately wanted to throw up, but remembered Dr Makker telling me to control myself. So I did. But the thoughts were more difficult to control.

Will I be able to survive six months of chemo? Dr Makker seems to have more confidence in my strength than I have in mine. Is she right?

The doctors had warned me that my second round would be the toughest and I would have to bear it stoically. I had been told that the liquid would fill up my stomach.

When the medicine dripped into me, I felt like a river of hot and cold was entering my stomach.

By the end of the session, my tummy felt stretched and ready to burst. Even sitting in the cab on the way back home proved to be painful. In my mouth was an acrid, metallic taste that refused every food my mother diligently tried to tempt me with.

In fact, the very sight of food began to make me feel nauseous. Any smells drifting into my nostrils made me want to throw up, but I controlled myself, keeping in mind Dr Makker's advice.

Mom wore a worried expression one day. I was supposed to walk every day, but I had not been doing it.

My mother explained to me that I must walk. 'Come out, Dad is waiting.'

Weakly, I hid my face inside the blanket. 'Ama, I can't walk.'

As if on cue, Dad appeared, ready to help me.

I can argue with my mom, but never with him.

He came up to me and gently pulled me to my feet. They felt wobbly.

'Come on, Manisha! Get up. Just one step, try one step. Now you can take another step. There, see? You can do it. Just walk up to that plant.'

'No, Dad. It's too far.'

'Just a few more steps. Slowly, one step at a time. Good! Now let's walk only up to that plant at the end of the hallway.'

My feet felt like jelly. I could not feel them. But I also could not refuse Dad.

'I'll hold you.'

Surprisingly, I managed to walk up to the plant. I stood still there, drained with the effort.

'Now stand next to this plant, Manisha. Take a few deep breaths. Phycus is among those plants that releases a good amount of oxygen.'

A smile curled at the corners of my lips. It must have been very difficult for Dad to express his emotions. He had always been a man of few words and a reservoir of unexpressed emotions. My mother used to tease him about this, coaxing him to say 'I love you' to her. And not rest until she succeeded.

I was very happy to see this tender side of Dad. I loved him more for the effort he had taken to break his self-imposed barriers. He had succeeded in getting his beloved daughter to do what he thought was best for her health.

My progress was slow. First a few steps in my bedroom, then my living room, then a few rounds of it and then into the corridor. This was my routine after every chemo session. Each dosage would bring my strength back to zero. I had to struggle to get it back up again.

I was very weak but Dad insisted that I take daily walks in the corridor of our apartment building. Looking back, that tender scene of my father helping me walk will remain etched in my mind.

Gradually, I could walk around the small garden outside my apartment, then a few blocks, until one day I managed to walk alongside the river!

* * *

Back in the apartment, Mom went fully into Annapurna mode. In Hindu mythology, goddess Annapurna is the incarnation of Parvati, wife of Shiva. *Anna* means 'food' in Sanskrit and *purna* means 'filled completely'. Annapurna is thus considered the goddess of the kitchen.

Mom was armed to the hilt with information gathered from my *nani,* an expert in home remedies, and her scientist and doctor friends. She decided that it would be only pure, unadulterated nourishment that would go into her precious daughter's body now! She had donned the same avatar when my father had fallen sick many years ago. She had rested only after he had bounced back to health completely.

Once again, Mom became a woman on a mission. After waking up at 3 a.m. and doing an elaborate puja, she would launch into her task of preparing something she was certain would make me strong again—Paya soup made of goat hooves. To this she added ginger, garlic, garam masala and fresh cinnamon. The concoction would take nine full hours to prepare, as she lovingly slow-cooked it so that I got its full benefits.

My mother is a doctor in the kitchen. She instinctively knows what to do whenever I have a pain, ache or any other problem. She learnt the art of healing naturally with food from Nani, who is an expert in the area of nutrition. My mother also meticulously planned my schedule based on the precious knowledge passed on by my grandmother. My mother excels in carrying on this tradition. To back up her knowledge, she takes the advice of her scientist friends.

This was my diet: a cup of turmeric milk in the morning; a hot breakfast consisting of two eggs, muesli with dry fruits and a little bit of milk; freshly squeezed pomegranate juice in the mid-morning; mutton soup, fish, vegetables, saag (greens), beans and rice for lunch; and beetroot, carrot and apple juice or fruit in the evening. Dinner was a regular meal, followed by turmeric milk before bed. When she first handed over the milk to me, she said with a lot of glee that she had added curcumin to it. I knew that she had spent hours slow-cooking this milk to get the full benefit of turmeric. My father had read in Dr Andrew Weil's *Guide to Optimum Health* that organic curcumin had anti-cancerous properties.

Mom began sourcing everything she heard was good for me. She managed to get the soft hilsa fish from her Bengali friend Dr Mukul Singh and asked my friend Avinash to get custard apple and ramphal (bell fruit, dadam or berry fruit in Hindi) as she had heard that it contained strong anti-cancer properties. She's a woman who will not rest until she has had her way.

But she is also like an enthusiastic, innocent child. One afternoon, she rushed into the apartment, her face bright with enthusiasm. She had asked her taxi driver—a Sikh man—to take her to the Queens area to buy Indian spices at the grocery store. Hearing that she needed groceries to provide me nutritious meals during my chemo breaks, the kind cabbie had invited her to his home. She had gone to an Indian grocery store from there and shopped for all the Indian and Nepalese items she missed sorely in New York.

From there the cabbie took her to a Sikh gurudwara where, much to her relief, everyone said that they would pray for her daughter and she would definitely get well. In gratitude, Mom stayed back to do seva. She made tea and rolled out rotis for all. This had been the perfect day for her!

With so much happening to ensure I became strong and healthy, I felt emboldened to face my next sessions of chemo. Soon I learnt, however, that being brave is only half the battle won. The chemo journey, like life, is dotted with unimaginable pitfalls and surprises that test your nerves.

I faced many roadblocks during my treatment. It started with urine and gum infections. I realized then the importance of maintaining the highest quality of personal hygiene during chemotherapy. Later, the catheter attached to a port in my abdomen got blocked due to some tissues and a surgery had to be performed to replace it. Just before the operation, one of the nurses asked me, 'Do you have any wish?'

Promptly I replied, 'To have a successful surgery and get my catheter implanted.'

My wish came true. After six hours I woke up to find that my operation had been successful. I had a big smile on my face when I was wheeled out and made to sit in a cab to go home.

One of the major side effects of chemotherapy is that, while chasing the rogue cells, it also kills the white blood cells in the body—the very cells that are supposed to guard you from illnesses.

But during one of my sessions, my white blood cells plummeted so low that it became a matter of huge concern for the doctors. An emergency injection was administered immediately.

How can I ever forget the pain of this injection? A long, pointed needle was pushed deep into me in a bid to awaken my bones. It was meant to nudge them to begin producing white blood cells once again.

I cringed, as the pain shot through me like fire. Colourful spots danced before my eyes.

My bones began to hurt badly. Bhai hurried over towards me and said in a near-scolding voice, 'You are giving up now? How can you? You are a fighter! FIGHT!'

The bone pain I experienced after this injection was unlike anything I had felt before.

Realizing my agony, my brother sat down next to me and pressed my legs lovingly. He continued to do so for several hours, as if he wanted to press the pain out of my body. I was grateful for his loving care, but the pain didn't subside. It felt as if someone were hammering me inside constantly.

The end result of this torture, however, turned out to be positive. I began to appreciate the tiniest of miracles that came my way.

To be truthful, despite all the discomfort and grumbling, after undergoing many sessions, I was fast becoming a veteran. I tried to handle the chemo sessions maturely, without unnecessary drama. I focused on finishing the entire procedure fast so that I could be done with it.

Just when I thought we were progressing steadily, one day I was refused chemo. I was hugely disappointed, as this would significantly put me back in my schedule. I remember feeling crushed when I was told that my platelet count had dipped so low that it was not advisable to go ahead with my chemo session. I was told to go back home and rest for two to three weeks.

Fear, disappointment and frustration swept through me.

I went over to the nurses and doctors and pleaded, 'Please let me have my chemo!' They remained unmoved, quoting protocol. So, with a heavy heart, I resigned to a three-week break before my next session.

But what about my survival? Hadn't Dr Chi stressed the importance of getting chemo on time? The right dose at the right time?

'Please, do not refuse me chemo!'

I was surprised at the passion with which I kept begging the nurse on duty. While people usually run away from chemo, here I was, begging for it. My mother looked at my disappointed face and, like always, came up with a solution.

She would get me to chew young papaya leaves. This, she had heard, was the miracle solution for getting platelet counts to shoot up. But the problem was finding tender young papaya leaves in the midst of a New York winter!

Frantically, Mom called up her friends in Mumbai and asked if anyone were planning to come to New York. They were all ready to do their bit to save my life. They would get not only papaya leaves but the entire tree, if Mom desired. There was one hitch, however. An unforeseen one. The Department of Agriculture and the Transportation Security Administration (TSA) considered it illegal to allow fruits and leaves from other countries to pass through customs.

Mom was stumped.

I didn't want to see her in such a situation.

So I contacted Naman-ji of Oneness University located in Varadaiahpalem, Chennai. The founders of the university—Sri Bhagavan and Amma—are believed to be divine avatars. According to Bhagavan, the university was created for just one purpose, 'To set man totally and unconditionally free, bringing about the Golden Age of Enlightenment.' I have been going to this sacred place in search of peace, tranquillity and divinity.

Naman-ji, despite being a spiritual guru of repute, is a brother to me—affectionate and dependable. Regardless of how busy he is, he always responds to me in a crisis. His parents had wanted him to be a chartered accountant, but he donned the white kurta-pyjama of spirituality and announced to them that his path and destination was god.

As usual, he gave me wise counsel. After listening to my fears, he simply said, 'Pray deeply to the *padukas*.' I had the silver footwear or padukas that I had brought along with me from India. They were considered powerful. You had to pray earnestly to the padukas, the feet of the divine, to connect. I did that.

To my delight, my prayers worked. Just a week later, I discovered that my platelet count had indeed become normal enough for me to get on with my chemo session. Excitedly, I lay down on the narrow hospital bed, eager to get on and be done with it.

During my chemo sessions, I started psyching myself into thinking I was getting vitamin shots, as Zakia had suggested. I looked at the inverted bottle on the IV tube attached to me as if we were old friends.

'This is a vitamin shot, not chemotherapy. Vitamin, not chemo. Vitamin . . . Vitamin . . . Vitamin . . .'

Once in our apartment, my desire was only to be with myself. I wanted no human contact. I became disinterested in what people were saying and confined myself completely to my room and bed. I was in non-thinking mode, suspended between life and death.

* * *

As the days rolled into months, and I continued with my chemo sessions, I hoped against hope that nothing untoward would occur. As the sessions progressed and the side effects of chemo took over, I turned into a dull, defeated person. The fear of death and the oncoming session of chemo began to loom constantly over my head.

There was a constant buzzing sound in my ears. I felt disoriented all the time. Like someone lost in a deep forest. Like someone who did not know where she was meant to go. Worse, like someone who did not know who she was.

Lying long hours on the bed, waiting for the chemo drips to chase the deadly villains out of my body, I went through every emotion possible—the excitement of coming closer to the finish line, pride at my own strength, the desperation at realizing that I may perhaps not survive it, the exhaustion of being ravaged.

Whenever I looked at the eyes of patients sitting outside, they seemed dead and defeated. With a jolt I remembered having broken my own promise to myself. I had resolved to not become like them. But I had. With great effort, each time I was photographed, I would enlarge my eyes to show I was still alive.

I had taken on self-healing as my pastime. Besides chanting Louise Hay's visualizations and affirmations for healing, I also started talking to my body.

One day, when Mom walked in, she was shocked to hear me speak in a voice that dripped honey, 'Beloved, you've done such great work looking after me. You've been through such a massive surgery, yet you are serving me beautifully. I know that you have the intelligence to heal yourself. Please guide me on how to look after you better.'

Mom was startled.

'Manu, who are you talking to?'

'My ovaries.'

'You're talking to your ovaries?'

'Yes, Ama. They've taken my ovaries out. But they still need my love. I'm also talking to my stomach and all my remaining organs. I am sending kind messages and gratitude to them.'

Mom went outside with a worried look on her face.

'Prakash, our daughter is saying strange things!'

At night, I would chant the Gayatri Mantra. I would also do the tulsi mala japa a thousand times.

As if one possessed, I kept on repeating the autosuggestion I had heard works on patients. I would look into my eyes in the mirror and say: 'I'm cured, I'm strong, I'm healthy, I'm fine, I'm cured.'

I was bent on not letting anything steal my rightful claim to positivity and abundance in health. I felt lucky. I had the best doctors looking after me in the hospital and the best Mom and Dad at home.

It was crucial that the chemo sessions ahead should go smoothly and uneventfully. But when has life followed our heart's desires?

The next bump was lurking just around the corner.

* * *

It was a cold winter night in the middle of my treatment cycle. I felt unnaturally weak and feverish.

It was 4 a.m. I debated with myself. *Should I wake up my brother?*

'Bhai, wake up,' I whispered softly to him. He was sleeping on the couch. I did not want to disturb my parents' sleep.

He looked up at me, confused and worried.

'Can you take me to the emergency please?'

'Now?'

'Yes.'

Sensing the urgency, Bhai immediately got up from the couch, ready for action. In the freezing dawn, we headed towards the emergency.

Have you ever been to a hospital at this hour? I had not. Its eerie sight startled me.

There were fewer people, and they all looked forlorn, their tired eyes staring at the walls. Some people had come directly from the station to the hospital, along with their luggage, hoping to get admission. I also noticed some women who were unescorted. They seemed to be really sick, but why were they alone? For a person like me, who had always taken pride in falling back on my family whenever I was in need, this came as a sad revelation.

I was told that my fever was the result of a urinary tract infection and that I had to get admitted immediately.

Not again, please!

To my great disappointment, I was quarantined and put in a secluded room.

The nurses strictly instructed everyone to not come near me without an apron and gloves. I had heard that a young girl, her immune system compromised after chemo, had died due to multiple organ infection. Alone and frightened, I could literally visualize viruses attacking me. Did the same fate await me as that girl?

What was happening to me? Was I also going to succumb to death?

I had to stay imprisoned in that room for three long, lonely days. My parents were not allowed to visit me during my quarantine. Both of them had a cold at that time. For fear of passing it on to me, they remained in the apartment, taking medicines for it. After three days, when my infection healed, I went with Mridula Di to New Jersey, which was one or two hours away from the hospital. Here, we were offered a stay at Kumi Aunty's apartment. Kumi Aunty is the late Vinod Khanna's sister and was Shail Mama's rakhi sister. I remained there with Mridula Di for 3–4 nights until I had completely healed. Once my parents responded to the medicines they were taking for their cold, I went and rejoined them in our New York apartment.

* * *

On one of the days during my hospital stay, Zeena-ji visited me. This time, she saw me not as the calm and collected woman who had been strong despite the bleak reports, but as someone who looked defeated and distressed. She continued visiting me each day, spending long hours with me. I asked her one day why she was doing all this for me.

'So that someday you will do the same for somebody else.'

In that moment, our relationship progressed from just a patient–visitor to that of soul sisters. Her husband, Dr Narula, was also my rakhi brother. I was grateful that I could reach out to them at any time of the day or night for support.

My equation with my family changed permanently through the course of my treatment. Our roles reversed. Earlier, I had been the decision-maker and caretaker. Now it was them. I felt blessed to have them around me.

During one of my chemo cycles, while I was sitting in front of Dr Makker, she noticed that I was on the point of disintegration.

She had concern in her eyes. Listlessness was visible in my stance, my voice, my eyes.

'Why don't you step out, Manisha? The weather is getting better. There are parks, libraries and gardens with flowers around. Go to Central Park. Go to New York Library. Go to a Whole Foods store and educate yourself about healthy eating.'

In a small voice I told her I was afraid of contracting infection.

Seeing me look like a frightened child, she melted. 'Don't be afraid, Manisha. I'm here. I'll handle if anything happens. Being stuck in a room, you're shutting life out. Go out, enjoy the little things, invite some happiness in and your chemo will become more effective. Leave the worry to me.'

My self-confidence lay crumpled on the floor. How could I go to these places? But the universe has a way of sending you help when you need it most. There were caring friends like Zeena-ji and her daughter who took it upon themselves to walk me out of my dullness.

One day, while Zeena-ji was helping me cross a road, my feet felt shaky and my head spun. My face paled and my eyebrows furrowed.

'It's a simple task—one you've done a million times before!' I told my brain. 'Just put this leg forward, then the next, then the first one and continue this for about thirty steps.'

But my feet were wobbly. I had simply forgotten how to cross a road! Why was this simple, everyday task so difficult?

Yet my caring friends continued trying to restore my lost self-confidence.

Dr Narayan Naidu, an accomplished scientist, flew all the way from the West Coast to the East Coast to boost my self-confidence. He would lighten our moods by taking us out for dinner and engaging us in deep conversations about spirituality and his journey. I was pleasantly surprised that a top scientist like him had a spiritual side to him. He gave me a lot of hope and became a strong rock for me during that period. I feel deeply indebted to him.

When Dr Makker asked me lovingly to take in some fresh air from outside, I felt like a lost child who had been reunited with her family. Dr Makker was kind, warm, compassionate—and caring!

Soon, I became close to her. One day I asked her why she had been so aloof, knowing my fears. Very gently she explained to me that this was the best way to be. She had adopted this approach because often patients became overly dependent on her and then, when they went away, it became emotionally difficult to snap ties. I looked at her with understanding and admiration. I soon began to see the affectionate side of my doctors.

* * *

It had been a particularly painful and exhausting chemotherapy session that day. I felt drained. Feeling trapped and at the end of my tether, I opened my eyes weakly to find Dr Chi holding my hand in his. His eyes said that he could read every thought in my exhausted body. He smiled his special kind of smile that radiated compassion and understanding. At that moment, he appeared to be god incarnate to me.

Soundlessly, without forming words, I said: *Doc, I have followed your advice as much as I could. Can you now tell me if I will live for long? I feel like my brain is running on 2 per cent battery.*

I felt he heard each word I had meant to say.

I closed my eyes, tears streaming down.

Outside, the desolation of winter was giving way to spring. Trees and flowers were waking up after their long sleep. Nature was rejuvenating herself. Everything was new and alive.

When would spring come into my life?

Would it ever?

12

Cancer-Free

'Feelings are like chemicals; the more you analyse them the worse they smell.'

—Charles Kingsley

With each chemo session my cancer markers started coming down. Zeena-ji and Jagat-ji, meanwhile, did my gene mutation test and discovered that I was BRCA-positive. This meant that I was susceptible to other cancers too. When I was told this, I sobbed the whole day, feeling sad at my destiny.

Knowing my emotional state, Zeena-ji came to visit me the next day. She informed me that her experience of working in the Lung Cancer Lab had made her realize that patients with mutated genes lived longer. While being BRCA-positive increases the chances of getting cancer, the good thing is that chemo works very well on them. That was the secret of my cancer markers falling so rapidly.

A piece of good news suddenly came my way. Instead of six months, my chemotherapy was now getting reduced to four months—April, instead of June. The reason was that I had responded well to the treatment. My heart soared.

This was *manna* from the heavens.

My body had been battered by four months of rigorous chemotherapy. Thirtieth April 2013 was the day of my last chemo session. Until then I had felt like a soldier who had injured his unarmed body and was debating which was better—to live or to die peacefully? But now life was showing me a tantalizing promise.

Spring was giving way to summer.

Soon, people would be out frolicking in the flower-decked parks, soaking in the sun and celebrating life.

Should I dare to dream that I will be among them?

In a fit of generosity, I said to myself: *Of course! Go ahead and dream. You deserve to after what you have been through!*

But I could not be too certain yet. All I knew was that I needed my cancer markers to become zero.

I decided to pray more intensely, deeply and strongly.

Like an impulsive child, I sought Dr Chi out and asked him with a big smile: 'Dr Chi, is it possible for the cancer markers to become zero?'

'You should not be worried.'

'No, no,' I argued, 'I want them to become zero!'

He laughed merrily. He was empathetic, very approachable and responded to the silliest of questions. My bond with both Dr Chi and Dr Makker had become very deep as we spent a lot of time together. I had got to see their warm, human side and felt immensely indebted to them.

In the days that followed, I remember praying fiercely to the divine. My silver padukas became my lifeline.

'Make my markers zero. ZERO! ZERO! Do you hear me?'

Almost like a wish fulfilment, my cancer markers dropped from forty to an impressive nine. But a perfectionist at heart, I refused to let go.

I kept sending frantic prayers to the one above and chanted like an obsessive woman. 'Zero! Zero! Zero!'

A few days later, magically, the count dropped to five.

Smiling and his eyes crinkling, Dr Chi told me that it was quite unusual for the markers to go below five.

Yet, having reached so far, I refused to give up. 'Zero! Zero! Zero!'

I could well have been an avid watcher of the Sensex in reverse.

I began chanting a lot. I would start the day with three japa malas. I would then chant the Surya Mantra. I followed this up with reciting the Oneness Mool Mantra 108 times during the day. Slowly, I started adding more mantras, 'I am healed . . . I am healed.' I would count the 108 beads several times over. I would do it silently and sometimes loudly too.

During my morning walks I would take my mala and keep chanting, 'I am strong . . . I am strong . . . My immune system is robust . . . My immune system is robust . . . ' I was also doing a lot of positive visualizations during my morning walks. I would visualize a bright colour—like the yellow rays of the sun—smashing the green, spiky cancer cells into pieces. I would also look straight into my eyes in the mirror and keep telling myself, 'I am strong . . . I am strong.' I kept trying to feed my subconscious with healing affirmations.

At night, just before going to sleep, I would protect myself with the Gayatri Mantra.

I don't know what worked, but continuing their downward journey, my cancer markers now became a commendable three!

During this time, I was always looking up stuff and collecting information from many sources, including books on naturopathy, Ayurveda and homeopathy to become an informed patient. I was obsessed with finding out alternative ways of healing. So while we were getting the best medical treatment we also tried out everything that was good for my body. We were hands-on with my healing process. We were all overjoyed when the chemotherapy worked and the cancer markers came down significantly.

As an Asian family living in an unfamiliar country, it was difficult to try out everything we could. We experimented with everything that my close well-wishers felt would work—nutritional interventions, walks, watching light-hearted movies, japa mala prayers, visualizations, developing a strong bond with the divine and even acupuncture that we discovered in the naturopathic section of Sloane Kettering. Needless to say, I remain deeply grateful to all the prayers and the wishes of all my fans. They helped me bounce back.

* * *

I remember that day clearly. It was 30 April. I was waiting anxiously for my blood report.

My anxiety prevented me from sitting still. I got up and walked to the coffee shop nearby. My eyes fell on two cute little girls. They must have been around two years old and looked like twins. I looked longingly at them and at their lucky mother.

One girl, who wore a pink frock and a pink bow on her straw-coloured hair, was clutching on to a Cabbage Patch doll. The doll seemed chewed on, jumped on and rather ragged. But she held on to it with a lot of love.

Looking at me smiling at the babies, the mother said, 'Oh, she holds on to her doll as if she is holding on to life itself!'

Just then, her twin, dressed in a tiny pair of jeans and a yellow top, came near her with an angry look in her beautiful blue eyes. Storming towards her sister, she grabbed the doll and threw it on the floor.

Her sister began to cry so loudly that the mother had a hard time shushing her up. It was only when the mother pulled the doll in question from the little bully that the little angel felt comforted.

Holding it tight against herself once again, the girl smiled a gorgeous smile. All was well once again in her little world.

It was a simple scene I had witnessed, but one that gave me hope. The pink-frocked girl had been holding on to her doll as if it were life itself. And she had felt threatened that she would lose it. But her story had a happy ending. She got her doll (life) back.

I found the situation symbolic of what I was going through. In a strange way, I felt reassured that I too would get a happy ending.

My blood report would be given to me any time now. Would it make me smile? Would all be well in my world again?

I returned from my walk and went up to the women's section where I was greeted by a nurse who led me to Dr Makker's room.

Dr Makker had a big smile on her face.

'Congratulations, Manisha! You are CANCER-FREE!

13

Stepping Out—Fearfully

'I'm not bitter. Why should I be bitter? I'm thrilled to death with life.'
—Johnny Cash

I was cancer-free! The black cloud of the disease looming ominously over my head had disappeared. And I was finally leaving the hospital and flying back to Mumbai.

Shouldn't I have been celebrating and jumping with joy, much like Annie, my bubbly character from the 1996 film *Khamoshi*? The girl, delirious with joy, grabs a broom—bouncing, capering and warbling a song:

Aaj main upar,
Aasman neeche
Aaj main aage,
Zamaana hai peechhe
Tell me, O khuda
Ab main, kya karoon
Chaloon seedhi ki ulti chaloon?

Today I'm on top, the sky is below me
Today I'm in front, the world is behind me
Oh god, just tell me what I should do,
Walk in a straight line or walk backwards?

But no. It was not pure bliss that I felt. My head and heart were swirling with conflicting emotions. Nudging out the initial burst of joy were darker clouds of fear—the fear of recurrence (which was a high possibility) and the fear of restarting my life in Mumbai (which I dreaded doing alone).

The past five months had been draining—physically as well as emotionally. Did I now have the strength to rebuild, reinvent or reimagine a new me?

And what about my finances? They had been severely dented during my treatment. How would I manage? Being an independent working woman, I had never leant on my parents for financial support. How could I do so now?

I was in the bedroom of my New York home. Just before boarding the plane to Mumbai I looked at my reflection in the mirror and stared into the eyes of a stranger—so fearful, so unsure, so *different*. I had felt joy at my falling hair and bald head. It meant that the chemotherapy was killing my cancer cells. But the joy dissipated completely when I thought of my future.

How would I face people like this in Mumbai? They had known me as a beautiful, glamorous star with lustrous hair and confident strides. But now?

The image that stared back at me was of a frightened woman with battle scars.

To my horror, I heard a hypercritical voice in my head: '*Haww! Kaisi thi! Aur kaisi ho gayi!* (Look how she was! And look what she has become now!)'

Visibly upset, I grabbed an eyebrow pencil and pencilled out my missing eyebrows. Then I applied some eyeliner and prayed that it would create an illusion of eyelashes where there were none. For the first time, I realized how difficult it must be to fit in and look like the standard version of a woman.

The apartment was in a frenzy. My cousin was busy cleaning the apartment, while Mom was packing Dad's and her own clothes. I needed to do something to calm myself.

I packed five months of clothes, books and medicines. I picked a red jumpsuit to wear, to denote the celebration of a new life. Its comfortable fit calmed me. But the eyes staring back from my mirror did not. Hastily I covered them with sunglasses.

All too quickly, it was time to board an early afternoon flight from La Guardia to Mumbai. As if to demonstrate the finality of this brave step we were taking as a family, all of us pulled our clothes tighter around us after seating ourselves inside the plane. My father adjusted his Dhaka topi tight, my mother snuggled deeper into the confines of her shawl and I pulled the hoodie over my head in an attempt to cover my face.

My heart was thudding. I felt sure others could hear it.

What must people be thinking of me? No, no, I don't want to know.

I felt briefly comforted when the pilot emerged from the cockpit and greeted us warmly. He ensured that my parents and I were comfortable. I was grateful for his empathetic gesture.

But there were those stares to be dealt with—even in first class.

What if I meet someone from the film industry? What will they think of me? How will I handle it?

Suddenly I froze. My eyes locked with Hrithik Roshan's hazel-green ones. He was sitting just one row away. With lightning speed, I averted my eyes, pretending I had not seen him. But Hrithik would not let the moment pass.

Can he read my fears?

He seemed to know what I was thinking. Leaning over, he said with complete genuineness, 'Manisha, you are looking great. Your skin is glowing.'

Softly, I whispered, 'Thank you!', not really believing him, but pretending to and wanting to do so. Desperately.

I shall never forget Hrithik's kindness. It had been my first encounter with the familiar world of glamour. I had left it as a patient and was coming back emaciated, yet cured after fighting a five-month bloody battle. I looked different. But in the warm sunshine of his acceptance, I felt some of my fears fading away.

I reclined in my seat and began concentrating on the peaceful scene outside my window. I let my thoughts fly to Mona, my financial adviser in Mumbai. She was in the process of cleaning my Mumbai home, making it ready for our arrival. She had hired a housekeeping company to completely disinfect the house. With my immune system so low, I needed a shield around me—one that would defend me against bugs, infections and toxic people.

I snapped out of my fitful sleep with the in-flight announcement. Mumbai awaited us. And so did my new life.

The all-too-familiar anxiety attack gripped me. Darkness bared its claws at me.

Emerging out into the crowd of people, I felt choked and weak. My brave mom walked strongly ahead. Hoodie on, I hid behind her, holding her arm for support. My eyes were focused on the ground. Not once did I look at anybody's face. I did not want to see their expressions at all. I desperately wanted to reach my apartment.

Somehow, I waddled through the crowd. A huge sigh of relief escaped my lips as I got into my car and we sped home.

Feeling suffocated at being trapped inside me, Fear finally spoke out: *So that was not too bad, was it?*

Bravado popped out and said: *Next time it's I who will rule.*

The beginning is always the hardest, I told myself. How could I dream of a better tomorrow if I remained stuck in my yesterday?

I would just have to be strong.

14

Team Mumbai

'Encourage, lift and strengthen one another. For the positive energy spread to one will be felt by us all. For we are connected, one and all.'
—Deborah Day

Unconditional support is the most powerful force in the world. One that is beyond judgement, beyond imperfections, beyond tangible reasons.

As if the universe knew exactly what I needed at that point, it poured huge doses of it on me. I think I came to life finally within the comfortable confines of my Mumbai home.

Sparky, my feisty little dog, hurled himself at me as soon as he saw me. He wagged his tail furiously and his eyes told me how much he had missed me. While I was away, my long-time house help, Vaishali, had looked after him.

And then there was Mona. She had helped me quickly liquidate my investments to ensure I got them on time for my treatment. Before my diagnosis, she had not even been a close friend. In fact, in her typically blunt style, she had told me that she had not liked me earlier. I was charmed by her honesty. But cancer picks out and places in your inner orbit the most unexpected of friendships. Emerging as a true friend in my time of need, Mona had gone to great lengths to make my home spick and span. She had also kept an eye on my house help and trained her to maintain a clean and beautiful home. Mona ensured that the house-keeping company drove away every known and unknown bug out. I thanked her lovingly for her support.

Dad and Mom decided to stay back in Mumbai for three months to help me out. Three dear friends also flew down all the way from Kathmandu to check on me. I thanked them profusely.

And on their heels came others. For there were a few heavenly beings who swooped down on me to support, surround and shower me with affection. They were Sushmita-ji, Shailendra-ji and Samir.

Let me introduce you to each one of them, before I explain the daily routine they put me through and the role each one of them played in healing me.

The daughter of a senior army officer in Nepal, Sushmita-ji is a meditator. Despite the luxury she was brought up in, her heart soon sought spirituality. She is now a part of Pilot Baba's group. She discovered that she had an innate gift of understanding the intricacies of nutrition. She came into my life as a mother figure filled with wisdom, ready to take care of me with her nutritional skills.

Sushmita-ji's stylish perm and bright-coloured salwar kameezes did not make her look spiritual at all. But then the moment you looked into her eyes, you were struck by her soul's stillness—the spiritual *thehrav*. Years of meditation had left its mark on her.

Deeply spiritual, Shailendra-ji looked his part. With his flowing white beard and deep, all-knowing eyes, he seemed to be wisdom incarnate. He was a businessperson who one day realized that his path was spirituality. Life for him was not only about earning money and providing for the family any more. In his free time, he would pursue his study of spirituality passionately and deepen his understanding. He then spent years in sadhana and meditation. Shailendra-ji now teaches meditation in Nepal and has a beautiful ashram near Kathmandu.

Samir is a friend who, after getting divorced, became disillusioned with life. He soon turned to Osho and became his ardent devotee. He took to spirituality, philosophy and meditation and now his life revolves around these aspects.

Each one of them had specific gifts which helped in healing me. Shailendra-ji helped me with guided meditation, Sushmita-ji cooked nutritious food for me and Samir taught me how to meditate the Osho way. They were a motley lot—people I loved and felt amused by. Surrounded by such experts, I felt like a dull diamond whose only task was to shine brighter each day.

Before my delighted eyes emerged a powerful team—some from Kathmandu, others from Mumbai. I fondly called them my 'Team Mumbai'! Their simple clothes belied their powerful identities. They were all successful householders and business owners blessed with a deep understanding of the spiritual.

The mission of 'Team Mumbai'? Taking care of me.

Their agenda? Restoring me to good health.

Their time frame? Yesterday!

They put me into a regimented routine, each expert not allowing the other to steal even a moment of their scheduled time from me. My day was divided into strict slots. Each hour was meant for a different activity. Throughout the day my 'Nepali Joes' focused on detoxing me, strengthening my immune system and monitoring whether the previous day's discipline had brought in the desired effects.

This is what my day's timetable looked like:

- **Early morning walks**

  By now I had become an expert in walking. I used to walk every day with Shailendra-ji, Samir, Sushmita-ji and Dad. I had long passed that phase of walking just within the premises of my home. Even in New York, we used to form groups and take rounds of Central Park which was just a few blocks away.

  Here in Mumbai, I began discovering parks around Yari Road and its neighbourhood. There were about seven or eight of them. We would pick one park and take several rounds of it and then move over to another park to walk some more. We were a bunch of three or four happy people, taking rounds of the park, sitting down to meditate and simply being super positive.

- **Breakfast**

  Mom and Sushmita-ji loved cooking special food for me. I needed protein to recover, so they went to great lengths to ensure that I got protein in delicious doses— all vegetarian. Sushmita-ji would make moong dal ki rotis, vegetable juices and other delicacies to tempt me. Throughout the day, Mom would go in and out of the kitchen as she wanted to make sure that I got fresh, nutritious and tasty meals. I could see my body and my appetite responding to this pampering and smiling back in contentment.

- **Rest**

- **Yoga**

  My yoga teacher, Suraj, would come home to teach me. While practising the different yogic postures, he would ask me to close my eyes and visualize that I was on the ghats of River Ganga. I would instantly get transported.

  As a child, living in Varanasi, I had experienced the magic of waking up at the crack of dawn and witnessing the most spectacular sight one can imagine. The majestic banks of the Ganga would turn into a stage for a sacred sound-and-light performance. Pandits would offer the morning *aarti* ritual to the gleaming holy waters as shlokas rang in the air. Soon, more people would join in and chants of '*Har Har Mahadev*', invoking Lord Shiva, would grow louder. As morning ragas filled the air, I would, as a wide-eyed child, feel mesmerized by the dancing flames in the many-tiered earthen containers. Rows of pandits dressed in white dhotis would hold these swaying flames in their hands and keep moving the blazing lights in unison. Reflected in the waters, the swaying flames seemed like fairy lights. The piercing sound of conches would fill the morning air, combining with the heady fragrance unique to a Hindu puja ritual. Gradually, the sun would come out and the spectacular sound-and-light show would end. I remember my little heart tugging when people called out to Ma Ganga. I would miss my mother.

- **Rest**

- **Lunch**

  Awakened by my walks and spiritual practices, my body eagerly awaited lunch every day. How wonderful it felt to see the healthy, colourful spread of raw greens, pulpy fruits and crunchy nuts! The rainbow-coloured food seemed to assuage my heart and nourish my body.

- **Rest**
  Post lunch, I would take a nap. Once I woke up, my eyes would still be heavy with sleep, but my mind hungry for knowledge. That's when I switched on audio books and let their wisdom about healing seep into me. It was a blissful time for me.

- **Physical training**
  It was Mona who recommended that I take physical training from Vikram. Having suddenly become paralysed after falling off from a great height, Vikram had worked on himself until his own exercises cured him. He had then become a physical trainer to help others. Vikram's story inspired me greatly.

  I was the right client for him. He taught me the power of functional training that would help rebuild me. Dr Chi had forbidden any work on my abdomen for at least a year since it had been opened and stitched back. He had told me that it would take a year to completely heal and until then, I would have to be careful. So Vikram and I began religiously working on the other areas. As we progressed, I began to develop a deep regard for all healers on our planet.

  My thoughts resonated with the inspirational author Shannon L. Alder's words: 'If you were born with the ability to change someone's perspective or emotions, never waste that gift. It is one of the most powerful gifts God can give—the ability to influence.'

- **Pranayama**
  Early evenings were reserved for pranayama. I have not yet met a pranayama teacher like Shambhu Sharan Jha. Pranayama is the regulation of breath through certain

breathing exercises, which clear the physical and emotional obstacles in our body. As a result, prana, or the life energy, begins to flow within. Through regular and sustained practice, one can supercharge one's entire body and mind.

- ## Osho meditation
And then there was Samir. He carried his unwavering love and passion for Osho like a flag that fluttered non-stop. Samir's Osho meditation tapes were dynamic. It required us to loosen up and move with the music. Every time a bell rang, we would have to change course. At the end of it, we would sit down quietly, in our personal island of tranquillity. If not too exhausted, we would listen to a discourse.

- ## Meditation and discourses
I practised guided meditation under Shailendra-ji's supervision. He had helped his mother-in-law, a stage-III ovarian cancer survivor, heal through his discourses and deep meditations. As I closed my eyes to begin my journey into myself, I felt comforted. If that good lady had come out restored and healed, why wouldn't I?

Under Shailendra-ji's guided meditation, I would dip slowly into myself, until by the end of it, I was completely immersed in a deep mind-body-soul experience.

He would explain to me the concept of Sakshi Bhava: 'Sakshi Bhava means to stand witness to all the phenomena that is happening around us. Through the senses, the mind perceives our reality. Sakshi Bhava helps us to witness every thought, feeling and sensation without identifying with it.'

As his explanation continued, I would slip into meditation and his words would fade away. The last words

I would hear were: 'It stops generating craving and aversion towards whatever we perceive through the senses.'

In the evening, we would sit around as a family and discuss the various spiritual teachings. I would ask questions that were troubling me.

- **Dinner**
The day's activities helped in awakening my appetite and I looked forward to mealtime. Back in New York, I would eat eggs and maybe, a little fish. But now my body began protesting against being loaded with animal protein. My stomach began rejecting non-vegetarian food. So it was decided. My stomach's decision was final. I became a staunch vegetarian.

But the fatigue I constantly felt remained. I trained myself to ignore it. There were better things to concentrate on—the light-hearted jokes we engaged in as a family, the sharing of lovely memories sitting around in a circle, the joyful digging into the 'nutritious meal of the day', the delicious aroma from the kitchen and the soaring of the spirits when the house filled with laughter.

By bedtime, my body would ache with all the physical exertion of the day. My bones, especially, hurt.

Very lovingly, Sushmita-ji would press the exhaustion out of my body expertly with her therapeutic touch. She knew exactly how to relieve my body of the pain. She would massage me till I fell asleep. Later, she told me her sweet secret. She would keep praying while massaging me. I was overwhelmed by her kindness, love and concern for me.

Gradually, the anxiety that had become a part of my personality in New York began peeling away. Very much like the tightly clasped petals of a lotus flower gently opening to reveal its full beauty. My home was clean, my beloved Sparky was with me and I was surrounded by loving friends and my parents who were there to pamper me.

* * *

The highpoints of my day, however, were my early morning walks. Let me share my 'discoveries' with you.

I discovered that I loved waking up early. It opened a whole new world for me. I was startled at the bounties nature had laid out for my eyes. As I used to always travel by car, I had missed the beauty around me. This was undiluted joy.

Getting up at the crack of dawn, I would often walk in my terrace garden before going to the parks nearby. I would watch in complete fascination how the sleepy, tiny white petals opened out one by one on the dense dark-green hedges, how the morning light reflected on the perfect balls of water on the blades of grass, how the just-woken-up birds played their orchestra from various trees on my path.

Why had I not noticed so much of beauty before? Why had I not realized how green the area around my house was?

Mesmerized, I started paying attention to the various shades of green the grass sported, the changing colours of the sky, the sharp and sweet smells the breeze carried on its gentle breast, the secret holes in the banyan trees and the age-old etchings on the huge barks—the names of lovers who had perhaps never become one.

I enjoyed feeling the cool breeze on my face. I began to pay attention to what I had taken for granted before: the birds, the beauty of sunrise, the different colours in the sky, the different shapes of clouds. My nature walks quickly became discovery walks.

Excited, I sought out other parks to walk in. To my delight, I found there were many—all within walking distance of my home. Like a kid in a candy store, I was excited.

I loved the feel of the crunchy green grass under my bare feet. I had heard that the western name for this age-old tradition was 'grounding' or 'earthing'. Walking barefoot apparently allows the earth to infuse our bodies with negative electrons. Through the open pores of our feet, we can actually soak in precious antioxidants. It made me aware of energy flowing into my body.

And then there were Mumbai's marshlands. Grasses, rushes and reeds dominated these low-lying wetlands. But it is the birds I noticed—a host of both local and migratory ones. Most had flown long distances, after spending summers on their breeding grounds in Arctic Russia.

In the midst of my walks, I would stand still, admiring the water birds—the blue-grey herons, bronze-coloured jacanas, the red-billed ibises, yellow-billed spoonbills, the stunning white storks as well as the waddling yellow baby ducks. They seemed to be quite comfortable with other resident birds like kites, kingfishers, shikras and koels.

But it was the graceful pink flamingos that quickly caught my eye. I loved their elegance. I still do not know why these splendid birds stand on one leg, with the other one kept tucked underneath their bodies. But it offered a charming sight. I understood then why people spent so much time birdwatching.

One scene I witnessed during one of my evening walks will always remain etched in my mind. The sun was setting and nature's drama was in full glory in the multi-coloured sky. Two things happened at once. The music of birds rained down on the ground below and at just that moment, raindrops began falling from the sky.

As I hurried towards the shelter of my home, I noticed a bird with eight legs! I paused. What kind of bird was this, I wondered, looking at its greyish-white plumage, black edgings and orange-and-black beak. I still do not know which species it belonged to. All I know is that it was a mother. A loving, caring mother. She had puffed out her feathers, spread out her wings and was providing shelter to her babies under them. My heart melted. This was mother nature at her finest!

* * *

It was the month of July. Pillows of dark clouds moved restlessly in the sky. For some time, the Mumbai air teased our senses with the smell of approaching rains. Even the waves did their bit by rising high, dancing and thrashing around to the music of the strong breeze.

The sky turned grey. The first drizzle fell like a gentle whisper. Soon, the pearls of rain falling on the sun-baked leaves turned to a tinkling—much like the lilting sound of champagne glasses clinking. The scene changed dramatically as sheets of rain intensified. Everyone ran for cover.

With the first showers came that delicious scent of rain on dry earth. My senses were assailed by this favourite childhood smell. I had read somewhere that the word for it was petrichor. Its etymology fascinated me. It is derived from the Greek words 'petra', meaning 'stone', and ichor, which refers to the fluid that flows in the veins of the Greek gods. I found this description quite romantic.

Next morning, everything appeared to be bathed in rain. Mumbai was rejoicing. The first shower, like the first kiss, had taken it by surprise.

I loved the feel of the wet breeze on my cheeks and the freshness and newness around. I had begun admiring nature's treasures that were sprinkled around me. I began to venerate each blade of grass and each leaf I saw. I think this state is called mindfulness. It was bliss.

One morning, I walked in the rain. It was such a liberating feeling. The birds were running for cover and here I was venturing out!

As I was walking one day in a newly discovered park near my house, I noticed people turning back to look at me. Some even stopped their cars. This time I met their eyes. What I saw in them was compassion and support. On a street, a man stopped to let me pass and gave me a thumbs-up! 'Manisha Koirala, keep up the good work!' he shouted.

I looked at him with 'new eyes'—eyes that had been washed by nature's purity. My heart soared. Instead of hiding my face underneath a hoodie, I bravely made a victory sign with my fingers and called out, 'Yeah! We're alive!' Two humans had exchanged happiness—at a deep human-to-human level.

How soothing it felt to discover that people were not laughing at me or at my bald head. They wanted me to win. I had never seen this beautiful side of humanity before. Everywhere I looked, there were people ready to help me.

I started falling in love with life once again.

The brisk walk in the fresh air outside stimulated my appetite. I came home tired, but nicely so. I looked forward to my healthy meal.

As evening fell and the sun's rays tiptoed out of my apartment, I felt the day stretching and yawning. Outside my window, I could see the orange-kissed sky turning the birds into dark silhouettes. Soon, they would be lost in the darkness, but not before meeting their families and telling them stories about their day's adventures. Having done that, they would roost in the dark, their head tucked under their wings until dawn.

Every evening at this hour, satiated with activity, I looked forward to going to bed. I felt at peace. My body felt like a temple. My mind alive. Where was the space to regret?

I crawled into bed thinking how wonderful everyone and everything was. Never would I let negativity and stress enter my body again and become cancer.

I looked forward to waking up early the next morning. I knew I would wake up to the birds chirping, the church bells ringing and the call to prayer—azan—floating in the air and mingling with the sacred sound of ringing temple bells. I was thankful to be alive.

Yes, I was not in perfect shape yet. I did not look the way I wanted to—yet. But I was surrounded by people who loved me. I smiled as I slipped into slumber.

Yes, my most favourite people in life will always be those who loved me when I wasn't quite lovable.

15

Home to Kathmandu and Chaos Again

'Keep your eyes on the finish line and not on the turmoil around you.'
—*Rihanna*

Have you ever seen an ECG graph? The peaks, the valleys, the squiggles and the flats? Well, that's how my life has been. Always unpredictable.

It was August. I had regained health and was now excited to be flying home to Kathmandu. I had no plans about how long I would stay. As a child, I remember pressing my little face against the windowpane of the aircraft each time we landed at my magical kingdom. Wide-eyed, I would drink in the beauty of my mountainous country. From up there, I would try to identify Mount Everest but never actually could. They all looked the same from a distance—stately peaks wrapped up in white pashmina shawls. As we descended closer, I would fly out a silent thanks to these lofty guardians for protecting us night and day, in silent vigil.

Coming home was always something I looked forward to. As a child, I would excitedly see Kathmandu emerge slowly before my wondrous eyes—first the mountains . . . then the lush green hills . . . the rivers . . . the riverbeds . . . the forests . . . the cultivated fields . . . the rice paddy fields . . . the brick factories . . .

the plains. . . then the scattering of a few houses . . . and then
we would land! I have loved this feeling of coming back home.
My excitement at coming back to the place where my entire
khandaan lives will always remain. It is magical.

On our way from the airport to my home, I began reflecting
on the days gone by. What blissful days my growing-up years in
Kathmandu had been! I had lived in my grandfather's two-storeyed
house in Chabahil with a huge garden. Both my grandmother and
my grandfather were towering personalities. My grandfather, Shri
B.P. Koirala, whom I lovingly called B.P. Ba, was deeply respected
for having fought for Nepal's democracy. The house was always
teeming with people—often with as many as fifty to a hundred of
them at a time. I loved being surrounded by grandparents, uncles,
aunts, cousins as well as the hordes of admirers and party workers
that swarmed his place.

In this huge house, equality ruled—beyond caste and
creed. Nobody was considered inferior. Everyone ate together.
People went about doing the tasks assigned to them, dressed
simply, never boasting about their importance. Even people
who cleaned and cooked belonged to the families of freedom
fighters.

The person from whom I learnt gardening later became one
of the top leaders of Nepal! He was Bhim Bahadur Tamang.
Our kids' group would learn gardening from him. It was he
who taught me to how to grow roses, strawberries, asparagus
and other plants in that huge garden.

Encouraged to explore various hobbies by my grandfather,
I excitedly took to gardening, cycling and roller skating. I also
enjoyed simply lying blissfully on my back on the dense grass,
among the frisky rabbits. Another activity I enjoyed was picking
unripe apricots and wild white flowers that I would later weave
into garlands.

I came back to the present with a jolt. As we drove from the airport to our parent's home in Maharajganj, Kathmandu, I saw the open spaces and pathways where I had learnt to cycle without brakes. Sadly, the ugliness of modern construction had taken away the beauty of the eucalyptus-lined pathways of my childhood.

Nepal occupies vast spaces of my soul. In Kathmandu resides the soul of both Hinduism and Buddhism—ageless, limitless, throbbing and alive. Looking back, I realize what a privilege and honour it was to grow up as a Koirala kid. Whichever part of Nepal I go to, I am still identified not as a Bollywood actress but as the granddaughter of B.P. Koirala, the first democratically elected prime minister of Nepal. Widely regarded as one of the greatest leaders of Nepal, he was a staunch advocate of democratic socialism, which he believed was the solution to Nepal's underdevelopment.

I love Nepal for its riot of colours, sights, sounds and smells, its mystic energy and its spiritually rich environment for both Hinduism and Buddhism. It is also known as Shakti Bhoomi and Tantra Bhoomi. Nepalis pray to Bhairav, who is another form of Lord Shiva.

Kathmandu is the capital of the kingdom, situated in a bowl-shaped valley, which is an open-air museum of various ancient temples and shrines, golden pagodas and magnificent deities. It is a city of unlimited historic, artistic and cultural richness.

It has often been described as the 'Land of Temples'. In fact, an old Hindu text describes Kathmandu as the land of gods surrounded by beautiful mountains. A western visitor wrote some two hundred years ago that there are as many temples as there are houses and as many idols as there are people in this city.

Kathmandu's most famous and sacred Hindu temple complex, Pashupatinath, was just walking distance from my childhood home in Chabahil. Recognized as a UNESCO World Heritage Site in 1979, this iconic temple is the seat of Nepal's national deity, Lord Pashupatinath.

Some of my most precious childhood memories are walking along the banks of River Bagmati that runs between the Pashupatinath temple and the temple of Guhyeshwari. The sacred Guhyeshwari Temple is dedicated to Adishakti. The library around the temple area has over 600 books written by Nepalese historian, writer and saint Yogi Naraharinath in twenty-eight languages. This library was my favourite haunt as a child. Even now, I love spending time there.

Kathmandu has many other striking visuals: the architecturally grand temples with their tapering tops; Boudhanath, the white-domed, golden-spired stupa, which is the largest in the world; the iconic Buddha face on the four sides of the square, which looks out into the four cardinal directions, with the all-seeing Buddha eyes; the piercing eyes of goddess Kumari; the red borders of the temples; the sprightly girls with red tikas on their foreheads; the married women wearing red-and-green bead necklaces (*pote*) with the distinct gold pendant (*tilhari*); and the red fluttering 'prayer flags'.

The stupas represent the human body, almost all of them having seven steps representing the seven chakras (energy centres) of the body. The eye of the Buddha is the third eye.

Dassain or Dussehra has always been a festival I looked forward to. Our extended family members would visit our home. It was a time when we all wore new clothes and the children went from house to house, seeking the blessings of elders. In our homes, our elders would bless us by putting a tika made of sindoor, yogurt and rice on our foreheads.

I love Nepal's distinct culture. I have beautiful childhood memories of the Tihar festival during the month of Kartik. It is a festival that celebrates the divine association between humans and animals. On the first day of the festival, Kaag Puja (crow worship) is performed by offering food to crows on the roofs of houses. The second day is for Kukur Puja (dog worship), where we garland dogs with yellow-and-orange *sayapatri phool* (marigolds) and apply tika on their foreheads. On this day, even the stray dogs look resplendent with tikas on their foreheads and garlands around their necks. On the third day, cows and oxen are worshipped. The third day is also celebrated as Lakshmi Puja. Windows and doorways are decorated with bright-yellow and flame-orange garlands made of sayapatri and *makhamali* (*Gomphrena globosa*). In the evening, the goddess of wealth, Lakshmi, is worshipped to express gratitude for the blessings bestowed on the family. Oil lamps are lit in her honour. The entire city begins twinkling like a fairy land. The fourth day is 'self day', or self-worship day, where we worship the spirit dwelling in our own body. Those following Vaishnavism also observe it as Govardhan Puja. The fourth day is also seen as the beginning of the Sambat calendar year in Nepal.

The five-day festival concludes with Bhaiya Dhuj, popularly called Bhaitika in Nepal. Sisters pray for the long and prosperous life of their brothers by applying multi-coloured tikas on their foreheads and blessing them. It is a day that celebrates the precious bond between sisters and brothers. On my mother's side of the family, I am the only sister. Hence I eagerly look forward to this celebration.

One of the most fascinating traditions of Nepal is the worship of Kumari Devi, or Living Goddess—a young, prepubescent girl who is believed to be the manifestation of the divine female energy or Devi in Hindu religious tradition. She is also considered to be the incarnation of the goddess Taleju, or Taleju Bhavani. The word 'Kumari' comes from the Sanskrit word 'kaumarya' or princess.

The main Royal Kumari in Kathmandu (there are several Kumaris across Nepal) lives in a palace called Kumari Ghar in the centre of the city. Kumaris with godly attributes are selected from among the Shakya caste or the Bajracharya clan of the Nepalese Newari community. She is generally chosen for a day like Navaratri or Durga Puja. In the Kathmandu Valley this is a prevalent practice.

A Kumari makes for a spectacular sight. Devotees carry her along the streets in a golden palanquin during the Seto Machindranath chariot festival at Hanuman Dhoka Durbar Square in Kathmandu.

I was once fortunate to visit and pay my respects to the Living Goddess. I do not remember my age at that time—just that I was a young child. Amidst the smell of thick candle wax and musky incense she sat, looking impassively at her worshippers from a low silver throne. Her dress was a vibrant red and gold. Her garland of deep-orange marigolds offset her very pale skin. She wore her hair in a topknot and had the *agni chakchuu* or 'fire eye' painted on her forehead as a symbol of her special powers of perception. The floor around her was strewn with ceremonial rice, decorative metal plates, red tika and white, pink, purple and dark-red carnation flowers. One by one, the worshippers came up to her and sought her blessings.

All these childhood images shot through my mind's eye as we landed in Kathmandu and drove towards home. Even though the 2015 earthquake caused massive destruction and death, the natives remain happy and hopeful. For me, this country beats to an ancient rhythm—life itself. I may go anywhere in the world, but the Nepali in me remains intact.

Finally, we reached my parent's home in Maharajganj. It was in a state of disarray, but the feeling of being home was indescribable. I felt safe and joyful.

I'll take it easy now! Maybe here I can relax my strict regimen.

At this point I had started receiving requests to give motivational talks. I used to always hesitate before accepting speaking assignments because I suffered from stage fright. You might think that to be strange, as I was a seasoned actress by then. The truth is that I have always been comfortable before a camera. But just remove that camera and put a mike and an audience of a 100 people instead, all waiting for me to speak, and I will fumble!

In the glow of what I thought was good health, I realized I had lost my fear of public speaking. So I accepted two assignments—one in Kathmandu and the other in Kolkata. But during the flight to Kolkata itself, I began feeling feverish. However, to my surprise, I delivered the speech effortlessly and flew back home.

I still felt feverish, but kept thrusting it to the back of my mind. But when my fever increased, I panicked.

What had I done wrong? Had I overexerted my weak body? Was it recurrence I was facing? No, not again, O divine!

Fearing that the water in my parent's home had caused this, I moved to Bhai and Yulia's home in the same city. But despite the loving care they showered on me, I showed no improvement.

My aunt who is a gynaecologist then took me to the hospital for tests. The sonogram revealed some spots on my liver! I was horrified. MRI tests were advised.

The damn cancer must have metastasized to my liver! Oh, why did I take the risk of travelling when my immune system was still so weak? Not again. God, not again!

We shot out emails to Dr Makker and she responded immediately (god bless her!), requesting more tests. Once those were done, she asked for some more.

Can you imagine living with the fear of cancer having recurred for ten full days? That's the horror I lived through. The matter had become more complicated as my gall bladder had been removed and there was no bile production in my body.

Frantically, I checked my cancer marker and heaved a big sigh of relief. The level had not increased. Sonography finally nailed the problem. Jaundice! I jumped with relief.

Perhaps the hard, unsterilized water in my parent's home had brought about the problem. Or was it the raw salad leaves I had eaten? One thing was clear. My immune system was very weak and I could not stress it further.

I stayed on in Kathmandu until I gained a little strength and then flew back to Mumbai—alone. I wanted to take one day at a time to rebuild myself. I flung myself wholeheartedly into strengthening and recovering inside out. The jaundice scare had shown me that I could not take my health for granted.

By the end of January 2014, I flew back to New York for follow-up scans. Dr Makker looked at my scans and said, 'Don't panic, but there's a spot on your pancreas. Most likely this is not cancer. It was probably always there and we missed it.'

My head began reeling.

'Manisha, I can ask the radiologist to write that this is benign.'

She had just said that to calm me and because she knew me. But the radiologist did not do so. Radiologists are in no obligation to do so. He did not know me and just did what he thought was right. Once again I plunged deeper into my black pit of panic and sorrow.

I was still uncertain about the results of my next scan. My CA-125 blood test reports were fine. But I knew this was not the most reliable marker. I was asked to wait for three months before doing a CT scan to check the size of the spot. In that mood, walking on razor's edge, I flew back to Mumbai.

I was certain of the worst. Mentally, I kept thinking of the 'ideal place' to leave the world. My dream place would have trees, birds and open spaces bathed in the sunlight. I would take my last breath as the fragrant breeze stroked me goodbye.

But I tried to gather myself. In a moment of clarity, I reached a decision. I would preserve myself. My mantra now would be self-care, self-mastery and self-discipline. I would not let any negative thoughts come near me.

16

Vulnerability—The Chink in My Armour

'It has been said, "time heals all wounds". I do not agree. The wounds remain. In time, the mind, protecting its sanity, covers them with scar tissue and the pain lessens. But it is never gone.'
—Rose Fitzgerald Kennedy

Almost everyone who has been through cancer will agree that we always look for emotional anchors. Sometimes we find them, sometimes we don't. But it doesn't stop us from hoping. At this time, I too was looking for the same, and that neediness made me take some wrong decisions. One of them was choosing the wrong person to have a committed relationship with.

I chanced upon a few old pages from my diary:

I was emotionally vulnerable. I had no idea what awaited me. Without mincing words and being honest, while still preserving the identity of the other person (as I don't really believe in mud-slinging), I would like to elaborate. I do so with the intention of accepting my mistake and maybe sharing my learnings with those who might need to learn from my experience. When we are in a vulnerable state, we tend to face pitfalls.

I have invested a huge amount of my living hours on the wrong friends and the wrong man that I can't really ignore it any more. I simply cannot pretend everything is hunky-dory in my castle. It's NOT!

A deep bond is created when we give good-quality attention and appreciation to people. I long for such friendships now, where I can comfortably call someone and he/she runs to help me and NOT make a big deal of it, where I would be sure that I am priority no. 1!

Choosing a partner is the most important and trickiest thing in the world. I say tricky because it deals with our own ideals and expectations. Yet when we get attracted, how quickly we forget the core values that are essential for a peaceful, loving, long-term relationship! We start looking at reality with rose-tinted glasses, refusing to see its real face. Eventually, the truth hits us, but if you are like me—stubborn—it takes a long, long, long time to finally accept it has been a defeat of sorts. Hell yeah! By the time one has accepted the setback one has been battered emotionally, mentally and sometimes, physically.

I was so sure that THIS TIME god had taken pity on me and sent answers to my prayers by letting him walk through that door in March 2013. I could smell the aircraft on him as I opened the door of my New York apartment. He had come to drop a book my friend Mona wanted me to read. I was down with loads and loads of chemo and had a bald head and swollen face with no eyebrows. My eyes looked tired. I used to gaze at people with a stark and empty look. I had turned into what I was running away from—I had started to look like other cancer patients.

I wondered if I looked human at all. I could not understand why he was so kind to me. He was so good-looking—tall, broad shoulders, long hair. He seemed so strong, yet so gentle and kind.

He came a couple of times afterwards. We exchanged emails and he told me of a few alternative treatments that I could try if the chemotherapy didn't work.

He knew a lot about alternative treatments as he had tried and tested every possible option for his parents when they were unwell. He had talked to many people about the different cures available. He told me about a doctor in Germany who did some alternative therapy. He even went ahead and fixed up my meeting with him. All I had to do was fly down to

Germany if this first-line treatment—chemotherapy—did not work for me. He came in as a huge support to someone who needed it badly then.

I loved the way he said, 'WE will get past these days and come out a winner.'

'WE'? Who does that? Who has the time and inclination to visit a dying woman with old parents looking after her? No one! My own friends had more important things to do. The boy I had been dating then had no time and no money to travel to New York. Once again I had made a blunder by choosing a person who could not be there in my hour of need.

I realized that probably it was my fault. I must not be worthy of a responsible and committed relationship. I felt lonely and scared.

And that's when THIS man walked in, stayed for long and kept on visiting me. I started to wonder if THIS WAS THE GUY! I was attracted to him but did not feel worthy of such a charmer.

It all started with me ignoring the fact that he was IN A COMMITTED RELATIONSHIP. I only saw that he was so good! I wanted to taste a bit of what dreams were made of. I argued with myself that I deserved this dream. This Prince Charming had walked in at a time when I had only death to look forward to. I was ugly, yet he saw beauty in me; I was unlovable, yet he made me feel worthy of his attention. The truth is, I ignored all the signs and all the obvious facts.

I started to make this dream my reality as I wanted it to be so. We had become good friends during our New York days—exchanging emails, calls and texts. He was there to give me support during my weakest times—during my chemo days; when I was apprehensive about how I would be received at airports; when I was scared of a cancer relapse in Kathmandu after Dr Makker discovered a new spot on my organ.

Nine months of kindness and loving friendship later turned into a full-fledged relationship in November. It had been a few weeks since I returned from Kathmandu and I was alone in Mumbai. He became my sole companion to various hospital visits in Mumbai and New York.

Everything was going perfect until I started to ask about his other 'someone'. I guess this was the beginning of the end of this romantic saga. He started to lie when I asked him about it. He told me that they were separated BUT STILL CONTINUING FOR THE SAKE OF COMMITMENT. That emotionally there was a disconnect between them. He painted a very grave picture of their relationship.

But I began feeling doubtful. I wished that what he was saying was the truth. I had a failed marriage behind me so I believed him when he said that he was in an unhappy relationship too. I prayed he was not lying to me.

He came in as the protective alpha male who would comfort me. 'I will protect you from the world,' he would say. I felt like a child amid mishaps. Very vulnerable. The relationship was like that between a rescuer and rescued. As long as this was the equation, it worked, as the roles were very clear. But the moment I wasn't in that victim role any more, and wanted to be on an equal footing, things started to unravel. The only problem was, I was deeply in love with him.

When his betrayal became apparent it shook my world and the effect remains to this day. It's not easy to recover from a heartbreak.

Ironically, it was at this time that I watched Ek Mulakat, *in which my friend Deepti Naval portrayed the role of Amrita Pritam. It was a play about the unrequited love between the great poets Amrita Pritam and Sahir Ludhiyanvi, who were madly in love with each other but had other commitments and partners of their own. This play stayed with me long after it was over.*

Midway through the play, it struck me that somehow, my story was similar. My heart was breaking and I was moving out of the relationship. Mine too was a story about unrequited, unfinished love.

My aunt's words echoed louder in my head, 'Manisha, you're very lucky in your work, but very unlucky in love.'

I was in danger of falling into depression and had to save myself. Initially, this friendship had made me strong, it had helped me fight through the pain. At that juncture in my life, it was almost a godsend. My need to be appreciated at my lowest physical, emotional and spiritual state had been met. He had helped uplift me and given me strength to fight. But now it had turned toxic.

I was also constantly mindful of the fact that I had a 90 per cent chance of recurrence right before my eyes, and I needed to pull myself out of anything that was painful and toxic. I was scared of falling into yet another emotional drama-packed relationship. My marriage had ended on such a note.

Was there a pattern here that I needed to release out of my system? My antennae were up. I didn't want anything to bring me down again. My focus was to win in the race of life, and I just didn't have space or time for anything that would pull me back.

I knew that I was not even ready for a relationship, as physically, emotionally and mentally I was still recovering. I knew that I needed to pull myself together and get the emotional strength to protect myself. If I succumbed now, I would regret that there were certain lessons that I had not learnt even after cancer. I was clear that I wanted to unlearn the bad patterns of attracting drama into my life. I desperately wanted peace and balance in all spheres.

So I gathered my strength. My survival instinct took over and I decided to detach from anything I was not ready for.

It was the bravest thing I did. I had dealt with cancer and come out of it. But to deal with a broken heart on top of that was painful.

I wasn't going to ruin whatever was left. This new me who had been given a second chance at life and wanted to choose life over death knew that giving into an emotionally toxic relationship could ruin my health and make my cancer recur.

It is only when a moment becomes a memory that you realize its true value. My determination to not see him without his wife had sounded the death knell for our relationship. He wanted to continue the relationship the way it was going. My condition was that I wanted to meet him with his wife to see for myself if his marriage was really over. He never met that condition.

In the gentle light of forgiveness, I felt deeply grateful to him. Grateful for the lesson he taught me.

True, the experience broke my heart, but it also gave me an understanding of my self-worth. It nudged me towards honouring myself and sticking to my principles at every step.

After the turmoil of emotions I had been through, I suddenly felt a deep peace descend over me. I sighed. This sense of closure was beautiful.

The new me wanted to only feed her soul with what was good for her and bad for the cancer cells.

When every cell in my body ached to hold my love for him tighter, wisdom whispered to me—let go.

Herman Hesse, the German-born poet, novelist and painter, was so right when he said, 'Some of us think holding on makes us strong; but sometimes it is letting go.'

17

Birthing the New Me in My Sanctuary

'You can either ask the question or experience the answer.'

—*Sri Bhagavan*

May–December 2014

In the beginning of May 2014, I bought a one-way ticket to Oneness University in Chennai, Tamil Nadu. On 30 April, at my Mumbai home, I had organized a small anniversary party of having been cancer-free for a year. At this party, I had felt perplexed, hurt and disillusioned by the lies that had been fed to me about my relationship. I felt Oneness would heal me.

I had visited the university earlier, between 2005 and 2006, spending some two or three months there, but it was not enough to absorb and apply the lessons I needed for my life.

This time, I was determined to learn, confront and change for good. This determination made me stay there for six months amid the peaceful green expanse—seeking, discovering and surrendering.

Sri Bhagavan, a spiritual leader, along with his spouse, Sri Amma, started the global Oneness movement in the early 1980s and by 2008 was reported to have more than 14 million followers worldwide.

So here I was in Chennai, sitting in a brown Toyota van which I had booked through a travel agent. From Tirusulam, where the airport is located, the place I was headed towards was a two-hour drive.

I had travelled to the southern part of the country several times as we used to shoot a lot here. In the nineties I came here for Mani Ratnam's *Bombay*. During those days I had not heard of Oneness University.

This time I was coming to drop all my labels.

- Manisha, the Alcohol-Dependent One
- Manisha, the Unforgiving One
- Manisha, the Bad Picker of Dudes
- Manisha, the Drama Queen

I was in a hurry to find out answers to my many questions: *Why had none of my romantic relationships worked out? Why was I always on the receiving end of judgement and pain for being honest? Why was there so much drama and toxicity in my life? Why had all these negative thoughts not gone away even after the suffering I had been through? What other thoughts needed to be rinsed out of me?*

There is something peaceful and rustic about the landscape there. I felt almost meditative as the car sped past huts, dogs, fields, bicycles and small shops. I saw strings of white jasmine flowers curled around the long plaits and buns of graceful Tamilian women. The smell brought in memories from my childhood—of my grandmother adorning herself with its tantalizing fragrance. For a minute I closed my eyes, remembering its comforting smell.

I preferred this lush foliage over Mumbai's skyscrapers. I love the fact that art, culture and tradition are carefully nurtured here in every child, with classical dance and music being an integral part of their growing-up years.

Soon we were at the gates of the university. Everything about Oneness spells serenity—its huge iron gates, the glowing white marble temple within, the quaint buggy ride that takes one to the ashram, the well-manicured gardens and the endless green expanse. I already felt my soul opening up to receive.

Within the residential section of the ashram I met my teacher, Chinmai Dasa-ji. To me she appeared to represent the powerful symbolism of the place I had come to. She was dressed in a simple white salwar–kurta and her head was shaved. On her forehead was a tika representing Brahma-Vishnu-Maheshwara and Adishakti, the source of all creation.

Chinmai Dasa-ji looked powerful, yet gentle, ancient, yet young, and demure, yet strong, depicting how humans can express all these at once. At Oneness, Adi Parashakti is the name given to the force behind all creation and everything that exists. God then is the summation and transcendence of all that is.

She smiled at me and I dropped my guard.

'Today, just rest. We will start your process from tomorrow.'

Yes, that's exactly what I wanted to do that day. To rest. To wash my soul of the heavy dust of the city. And the heavy baggage of the mind.

My tiny room had many windows. I flung them all open to take in the sight of the whispering trees. I breathed in the fresh air.

It was late afternoon. The sun was a golden orb, setting in the distance. Just like animals lay territorial claim to their spaces in innovative ways, I did too. In my room, I arranged some of my favourite stuff—incense sticks and essential oils—on the table to personalize it. I unpacked some books too and decided to make it my writing table. I then laid out the precious items from Oneness I had picked up on a previous visit: the silver padukas, a japa mala, holding which I recited

the mool mantra, a small notepad, a book of other mantras and
most importantly a gratitude notepad. I was happy to see that
my room had Wi-Fi connectivity. It meant that my iPad and
phone would work.

I unpacked my clothes and hung them neatly in the cupboard.
Finally, I placed a picture of Sri Bhagavan, whom we call Srimurti,
on the side table beside my bed. I requested for fresh flowers to
be delivered to my room. I decorated the Srimurti with them,
lighting scented candles and incense sticks. I also placed a cushion
on the floor facing the side table to perform the daily puja. I
looked around and was happy that my room looked like someone
had moved in and planned to stay here a long time.

Soon, I was ready to sleep.

I woke up feeling very fresh and hungry. I walked to the
dining area and was happy to see rasam and rice being served.
I could not wait to swirl the ball of rice dipped in tangy rasam
into my mouth. Mindful of the deliciousness of each mouthful,
I realized I was participating in eating meditation. I love the
variety south Indian food offers. It is so pure, each mouthful
a burst of spicy tastiness. I ate some curd rice to balance the
delicious fire on my tongue.

After sipping chamomile tea which I had brought along
with me, I decided to walk on the green expanse barefoot,
mindful of each blade of grass nudging my soles and waking up
my soul.

Satiated, I walked back to my room. Sleep—rich and
peaceful—wrapped me in its serene arms.

I woke up the next morning refreshed and ready to learn.
Chinmai-ji walked in with a big warm smile and quietly led
me down to the marble white temple. Leaving me sitting on
the floor, bowing my head before the divine, she walked away
quietly.

Intuitively, she understood that all I needed at that point was some time to myself to process my feelings. I was grateful to be alone. People usually flock to Oneness University in the months of July and August and some come for a few courses in June. In the month of May, I was almost by myself. In June, people slowly began trickling in.

During May and June, the only inhabitants there were the management, the people belonging to the administrative department and the teachers at the university. There was no interaction with the few seekers who were there at that time. This suited me fine as I wanted some 'me time' and the time to connect with the divine. I was grateful for the serenity and tranquillity that came with being by myself there.

On the first floor, in the expansive meditation room, I soaked in the stillness and the energy of the place. I was not sure what I needed to do. So I sent out a silent prayer to the divine:

Please guide me in this process and help me discover if there is any toxic pattern I need to release from my system.

I was waiting for god to answer, but he refused to do so.

But I felt a sudden upheaval from inside me. Without warning, I let out a grief-stricken, primordial howl that emerged from my innermost being. It bounced off the ornate pillars, swept through the vast marble floors, brushed against the ancient trees outside and bounced back to me, lying limply on the intricately woven hay mattress I sat on. Tears flowed non-stop, rising from my innermost being. It was grief peeling from within several past lifetimes.

After around two hours, I felt spent, drained, exhausted. My wail had come from a space of deep sorrow.

I cannot afford to waste my life. I don't want to be in this broken state any
more. Help me! Heal me!

After two hours, the tears stopped. With that descended
a comforting peace and the resolve that in the months ahead
I would shine light into all the intricate, hidden dark spaces
inside me—into each layer I was hitherto unaware of.

I spent many months—most of 2014—there. In the
month of August I flew to Delhi to receive the India Today
Woman of the Year Award and came back to Oneness again.
In September, I went for a brief visit to Mumbai.

This is how May turned to August until September turned
to December. I was processing a lot. I was a woman on a long,
complex and never-ending journey.

There were no lists of dos and don'ts at the ashram. We were
each left to ourselves. But the discourses I attended left a deep
impact on my mind. These are Sri Bhagavan's basic principles:

> We are nothing but programs—programmed from previous
> lives, right from the time we were in our mother's womb
> to the hours leading to our birth, incidents leading to our
> life, events during the growing-up years, until our present
> emotional state. If the programming is unhealthy, we need
> to be mindful of unhealthy patterns.

I took a sharp breath in. Why was I programmed to attract
drama and emotional toxicity? 'Enough,' I shouted to the
universe. 'No more!'

To transform my life inside out, I would need to dwell on
every aspect of my programming. And that required me to be
brave.

After hours of meditation and deep contemplation, I
started digging deep into myself. Through the prism of my still,

seeking mind, I first examined my negative programming. 'We are nothing but programs,' Sri Bhagavan had said.

It was time to reprogram myself.

Manisha, the Alcohol-Dependent One

In school, I had always been a shy, introverted girl who found solace in books. I think reading a lot of books does that to you. I was ahead of my classmates in some ways. While they were enjoying Mills & Boons, I was reading Ayn Rand.

When films happened suddenly, I was just nineteen years old and not ready to handle Mumbai. Its unfamiliarity and expanse scared me. For a young, unexposed Nepalese girl, Bollywood was a terrifying experience. Unsure of how I should be behaving and interacting on the film set, I hid myself behind books. They protected me from my fear of interacting with everyone who seemed to be so sure of themselves.

My mother encouraged me to adapt, socialize and try to fit in. I remember the time Raveena Tandon and Somi Ali came home, all ready to plan a night out. I was reluctant to go, but Mom insisted that I make friends from the same profession and the same age group. Earlier, my visit to a female colleague's home for a few parties had left me feeling inadequate. She was bright and happy and came from a film background and had many friends in the industry.

I would look in admiration at my brother, who studied at Doon School, Dehradun, and had more friends in Mumbai than I. I decided to do something to overcome my shyness and feeling of awkwardness.

Alcohol came to my rescue. I loved the feeling of confidence it gave me, loosening me up, wiping out my inhibitions. Fortified by drinks, my shyness disappeared and I became quite at ease while socializing. Emboldened, I took to drinking more . . . and more.

Parties became a way of life for me. Either friends would party at my house or I would go over to theirs.

I realized how it had seeped into my life. I look back at that period with a lot of regret and sadness.

In Oneness we are taught to become aware of the unhealthy parts of our personality. Once you are aware, you begin working on it. Once you see that you were driven by unhealthy actions, you act upon them. Once you see the mistakes you have made, you change the course of action. You begin taking the right action if you were unaware that those that you took in the past were wrong. Confidence needs to stream out from within you, not from anything else. And you need to be comfortable in your own skin.

'To see is to be free'—Sri Bhagavan

Manisha, the Unforgiving One

An emotionally sensitive and charged person, I had been collecting and storing away every hurt, disappointment, anger and negativity deep inside me. As a defence mechanism, I would plaster the exteriors of these ugly beings with a pretty 'I'm okay' smile.

In the light of newly gained wisdom, I saw my body as a transparent glass container, stuffed with bruised, dark, injured and bleeding emotions. What were they doing in my beautiful body? So I carefully reached inside, picked up each one and examined them. Many had festered and pickled and were corroding my insides. One by one, I turned them in my fingers, snapped my ties with them and disposed them of far away where I could never reach them again.

I felt light and free.

I now delved deeper into myself and began to examine my friendships. Thanks to the strength and confidence-inducing power of alcohol, I had many friends whom I could call mine. My fun bunch was ever ready to party or fly over to Ibiza or Amsterdam at the shortest notice. We shopped till we dropped and travelled to our heart's content, wherever our fancies took us. I had a great time.

But now, where had all them disappeared? None of them came to visit me after I was diagnosed with cancer. Were our bonds not strong enough?

In the months ahead, I felt the hurt of their abandonment burning fiercely inside me. Lying in my hospital bed, I constantly asked myself, why hadn't they come in my time of need?

In this sacred space of understanding, I realized that fun being the core of our friendship, our relationship had disintegrated the moment the focus had changed. It was fun to meet a fun friend, but not fun at all to visit a suffering one.

My flippant lifestyle had left no space for deep bonds. But I could see things more clearly now. It must have been difficult for them to acknowledge the transformation of a 'happy party symbol' to a 'dejected, dying woman'. They wanted to hold on to that happy image of me in their hearts.

And now was the time to introspect. Had I been a good friend, worthy of deep friendship? My heart said no. Was I the kind of friend I expected others to be? Guiltily, I remembered my many transgressions.

At the late Divya Bharti's prayer meeting I had breezed in and left within a few minutes. Why?

The late Feroz Khan and I had shared a deep affection for each other. He was my favourite person in the industry. He had directed my third film *Yalgaar* (1992). How affectionately he used to call me Manish! His entire family knew how fond he was of me. Feroz saab had also shown immense love and respect to my family. Just before his death, he came back to his Mumbai home. Shouldn't I have asked his family if I could be of any help? Shouldn't I have visited him and spent time with him instead of paying my respects only at his *chautha* ceremony (the fourth day after death)? But I didn't. Why?

The late Ashok Mehta-ji was a friend, well-wisher and, moreover, a mentor who helped me pick the right films. He too had been struck by cancer. He withstood the attack for two years but then the cancer entered his brain.

His eyes lit up when he saw me by his hospital bed at Dhirubhai Kokilaben Ambani Hospital, Mumbai. But I felt dumbstruck. I didn't know what to say as this strong man's eyes filled up.

'Look what's happened to me,' he said mournfully.

'There! There!' I told him.' Don't cry! Be strong!' That's the best I could do. Shouldn't I have simply sat there and let him cry his heart out at the unfairness of it all? Shouldn't I have said, 'I am right here with you and will not leave you'?

Maybe we should have shared tears together. Shouldn't I have sat longer with him? But I didn't. Why?

When I thought of all this, the behaviour of my friends seemed immensely pardonable.

In my new, awakened state, I understood that like me, they too were uncomfortable facing pain and sadness, especially if it was that of someone who had been cheerful and fun-loving. A dying person is a reminder of our mortality. At some level, each one of us wants to avoid confronting our own mortality. After understanding this, my resentment vanished. I hugged them in my heart with deep compassion and thanked them for the fun times we had shared.

I forgave them as I forgave myself.

'External world is a reflection of your inner world.'—*Sri Bhagavan*

Manisha, the Bad Picker of Dudes

During the months at Oneness University, I finally picked up pieces of myself to examine my relationship with love.

But before that, I needed to make one call to get closure from my recent heartbreak. He answered me brusquely, accusing me of having loose morals. I was horrified. This came from a man whose morals were questionable as he had been married for long. Despite this and having a grown-up son, he had conned me into believing his sob story and promised me eternity. God knows how many other flings he might have had!

That did it. This was the death knell I sought to progress on my spiritual path. There was clearly a toxic pattern at work here.

Looking closely at my relationship with love, I saw how it had become rancid because of my neediness and vulnerability. My desperate need to be loved always made me jump headlong into it, without checking whether the person was mature and sorted enough to handle the relationship I wanted. And in all this I had overlooked the big basic question—was he even capable of living life with honesty?

The drive and need to be loved or find an emotional anchor had been my undoing. I had blundered by giving my wholehearted love to another without really knowing the person. My need to be loved had overruled my objectivity. Was I seeking the wrong reasons to be loved? Can need or fear of loneliness ever be a good enough reason?

I decided that I would never again seek another human being as my anchor. Instead, I would solidify myself.

I found 'aloneness' instead of 'loneliness'. There is a huge difference between the two. All + oneness is aloneness. I now felt comfortable in my own company. I discovered freedom from the need for a companion.

'Detachment cannot be practised, it must happen to you.'—Sri Amma Bhagavan

Manisha, the Drama Queen

As the months at Oneness passed by, I went deeper and further into myself, my discovery leading me to my life's core issues— patterns that had governed my life . . . the paths that had already been carved, willing me to walk on them like an unthinking puppet.

I was now discovering my true path of well-being, knowledge and spirituality. Infused with the emotional strength this produced, I was led to new realizations. I felt confident that I could now beat predetermined toxic patterns that had led to my cancer. I was now aflame with the desire to heal my emotional body. No more drama, no more toxicity!

A long time ago, I was asked to emote the pain of a mother looking for her two children who had gone missing on the streets of Mumbai. It was an intense scene for *Bombay*.

I was going through a difficult period emotionally in real life at that time. The pain of that became the source from which I drew my emotions for the scene. The audience loved it. That became my cue and my inspiration.

Was I unconsciously creating drama in my personal space so that I could pour my heart out into my roles? Was that the reason most creative people led stormy lives? Why do the personal and the professional borders blur?

I made the decision right then. I would no longer utilize the drama in my life for drama on screen. In fact I would avoid drama in my personal space as much as possible. Leading a peaceful life was what my heart desired. And self-preservation would now become my priority.

Life itself was exciting; adding drama was a trouble I could do without. In stillness and peace I could see the true beauty of life.

I had become my own roadway. I had become my own destination.

'In stillness of thought you discover oneness.'—Sri Bhagavan

18

Lessons Learnt, Wisdom Passed On

'Healing is a matter of time, but it is also a matter of opportunity.'
— *Hippocrates*

I have been a relentless seeker all my life. I am as curious as a beaver. As resolute as a woodpecker.

Now that I am healed, I wish to help others. I am curious to learn how I was cured so that I can pass on my learnings to you.

I was afflicted by stage-IV cancer that had metastasized. (Yes, it wasn't stage-III cancer as I had thought all along. I only discovered this when my lab results came out post the 10 December surgery.) I know many such patients who did not survive. Somewhere, I feel the survivors' guilt. But I push it down, wanting to rejoice in the here and now.

Knowledge is power and being forearmed means being safe. So let me step back a little and allow you to absorb the knowledge I got from my conversations with my two life saviours—Dr Chi and Dr Makker.

Below is an excerpt of my conversation with Dr Chi:

MK: In your experience what kinds of patients do well in late stages of ovarian cancer?

Dr Chi: There are multiple factors that can predict how well a patient will respond to treatment when diagnosed with advanced ovarian cancer. These prognostic factors include:

- Age at diagnosis. Younger patients do better than older ones.
- The subset within the advanced-stage disease. Stage IIIA does better than stage IIIB, which does better than IIIC and IV and so on.
- Whether or not there was a cancerous fluid called ascites during diagnosis [my stomach had bloated up with this fluid making me look heavily pregnant].
- The nutritional and overall health status of the patient.
- Whether or not there is a BRCA mutation in the patient or the tumour [I was BRCA-positive].
- Amount of cancer found at initial surgery and the amount left behind post surgery. Less is better for both. Less than 33 is considered normal [My CA-125 (a cancer marker) was as high as 600. After surgery it went down to 40 and after my chemotherapy it was less than 10].
- The mix of chemotherapy drugs used in treatment.

MK: Why do you think I did well?

Dr Chi: You did well because you are young and healthy with a good nutritional status. The tumour was responsive to surgery and sensitive to chemotherapy. You received state-of-the-art surgery as well as post-operative chemotherapy.

MK: What do you have to say to those who get diagnosed with late-stage ovarian cancer?

Dr Chi: The diagnosis of advanced ovarian cancer is not a death sentence. However, there are only two factors that the doctors or patients can control once the diagnosis is made: How much cancer is left behind after surgery and what type of chemotherapy is given. Hence it is crucial that once you are diagnosed with ovarian cancer, you have to go to a centre of excellence. You did that and got the most optimal outcome.

I also had a few questions for Dr Makker.

MK: Doctor, could you please tell me about my first chemo, the allergic reaction I had and your treatment for the same?

Dr Makker: On 8 January 2013, you were given an intravenous infusion following which you complained of stomach pain, heat, sudden nausea and lower back pain. The chemo infusion was then stopped.

We restarted your chemo approximately one hour later after we treated your allergic reaction and you tolerated the rest without any issues. You had a high blood pressure of 149/103 and a heart rate of 128 when the episode started which then improved to 110/80 and 100 when the episode abated. After this you were okay.

MK: Doctor, what is your advice to patients diagnosed with cancer, especially those with late-stage diagnosis?

Dr Makker: Manisha, my general advice varies depending on their stage and also the genetic risk factors.

We always try to bolster our patients' confidence as they learn of the diagnosis and also try to provide a great deal of emotional and psychological support [I can vouch for this as she was a great source of support during my treatment and after. She is the same with all patients.]. We also have social workers and case managers who provide a great deal of support.

A diagnosis of cancer and chemotherapy can be daunting, so we tell our patients to take things one day at a time and to focus on taking care of themselves (sleep, follow the right diet, be spiritual, exercise). We remind them that this is a marathon and not a sprint. We tell them to be proactive in communicating their needs. We also ensure that all patients get genetically tested so that we know whether there is a genetic predisposition to their disease. Further, we encourage patients to be well-read and educate themselves regarding clinical trials, especially in cases where the cancer recurs.

In terms of categories, we do that once the treatment is complete. We see how they are doing then. Patients who have disease recurrence within six months of completing their initial platinum/taxane-based chemo, that's the group we worry the most about, and it is this group that does the least well. But there is a great deal of work that is being done with regard to clinical trials for this population of patients and also for those with more indolent diseases.

* * *

I remember how Dr Makker would consistently urge me to step out and enjoy the sights and sounds of New York. She encouraged me to exercise and suggested some options for clinical trials as well. She is constantly in touch with her patients and replies to all my emails. She suggested that I get a doctor in Mumbai whom she can constantly be in touch with. Wherever

I am, whether in India or Nepal, Dr Makker makes sure I am doing well. Both Dr Chi and Dr Makker have set the highest benchmark for a patient–doctor relationship.

As for my questions, they continue to be numerous. Part of me desperately wants answers:

Why am I fine and why did my cousin, who was struck by cancer at the same time, pass away?

What is my role in this second chance at life?

Why did I get cancer in the first place? God dammit! Why couldn't my lessons have been less painful?

My questions might appear ignorant, but they are an attempt to understand life's deeper mysteries. They are born out of my journey of pain.

So the picture is clear. I survived because of all the support, medical expertise and my will power to do well.

Let this be a learning moment for all of us. Cancer can be overcome by making different choices, by being equipped with the right knowledge and having a solid support system. Unlike the Westerners, we Asians are fortunate to still have our family network intact to support us in crises.

The purpose of my book would not be complete without talking about the triggers that I feel were the cause of my cancer. I strongly believe that our emotions play a huge role in creating our reality. Emotional health is therefore crucial in keeping illnesses away. I am no doctor, but do indulge me while I play counsellor and analyse my life.

Lack of Gratitude

In the midst of my film career, while I was at my peak, I suddenly felt a deep sense of disengagement. I had everything and yet felt low.

Working on twelve films in a year, eighteen hours every single day, with three shifts in three different corners of Mumbai exhausted me. I could not handle Mumbai's traffic jams. I could not handle the fact that I was not allowed to explore the countries we went to due to shortage of time and my workload. I could not handle myself. Was it burnout?

Maybe, but I admit I was left with no gratitude for the blessings I had. I simply did not value my good fortune.

My Emotions

I felt chaotic, and my emotional life reflected that. I latched on to romantic relationships because I felt unhappy and unloved. Instead of nurturing myself, I began seeking out nurturers. Not only did I never get them, but they left behind a lot of toxicity which I had to deal with myself. I think this build-up of emotional toxicity finally made my body collapse.

Lack of Receptivity

Somewhere down the line, I had become numb. Numb to my own emotions and to that of my family's. I refused to listen to them. They saw me suffering, but I could not see what they (particularly my loving mother) were going through, seeing me in this state. I partied mindlessly and slogged mindlessly in my attempt to numb my own numbness. I was tired of my routine, of my heartbreaks, of the unforgiving paparazzi. Blind, stubborn and ignorant, I simply drifted along thoughtlessly.

Hormone Treatment

It hit me one day that I was about to turn forty. My body clock was ticking. I wanted babies desperately. But I knew I needed to get married fast. The man I was dating then did not see a future with me. So I dropped him and got married in a hurry. I badly wanted a home and children. It clearly was the wrong reason to get into such a sacred relationship. Much to my sorrow, it did not work out. When I felt it disintegrating, I thought perhaps a baby would make it work.

Emotionally, I was at my lowest then. Everything was going wrong. Why was my dream of a happy home collapsing? Yes, kids would save this marriage, I thought. I was not able to conceive naturally, so I went ahead and took IVF (In Vitro Fertilization) injections. Little did I know what havoc they would wreak on my body. I was BRCA-1 positive. Was it the injections that triggered my ovarian cancer? I would never know for sure as this has not been proven medically.

Wrong Lifestyle

For a decade, I had abused my body. The poor lifestyle I had been leading made my body susceptible to diseases. Had it not been cancer, some other malady would have struck me. In hindsight, on a dark, lonely night, I still wonder what it could have been and whether it would have been better or worse.

Emotional Turmoil

I have always been an emotional person, ruled by my heart and not my head. The shame of previously failed relationships was enough to make me want to make my marriage succeed. But I was also ignorant of the ways of the world. Looking back, I kept asking myself many questions.

What if I had responded differently to that argument? What if I had done the expected thing then? What if I had not been drinking? Would I have still got married had I known a nightmare awaited us?

The ifs kept going round and round in my mind like a giant Ferris wheel. But, as is always the case, one's hindsight is always 20 by 20.

My experience has made me wiser. To all those women who feel stuck in their relationships, I have a piece of advice. Try as hard as you can, but if it seems like a situation beyond repair, please do not suffer silently. Don't let societal shame or pressure keep you tied to a situation. Ask for help. Reach out. If you keep on enduring it silently, your body will become a host to potential diseases.

None of us know why some of us get cancer and others don't. None of us know why some succumb to it and others recover to tell the tale. All I know is that I am one of the lucky ones and will use my life to help other women who need to learn from my experience.

I shall continue reading and seeking more answers from those who are learned or knowledgeable. And I shall continue appealing to people to change their attitude towards cancer. I feel angered by the way people treat those afflicted by it.

I remember a poverty-stricken mother telling me how her only child had been ostracized by her community after he was diagnosed with cancer. All sorts of stories began floating around, including that everyone should stay away from the 'infection'! I want people to stop shaming those who have cancer or telling them that it is all due to their karma or past sins. All this is hogwash and nobody has the right to pass judgement on anyone afflicted by it. It is not only cruel, but criminal to do so.

Medical science is still trying to uncover the cause of cancer and it's cure. Until then, let's look after our bodies well. Let's give it the gift of healthy nutrition and a balanced lifestyle.

Let's be compassionate to the stricken. Let's spread hope. Let's heal each other through love and kindness. God knows the world needs more of that!

19

Cancer as My Gift

'A scar does not form on the dying. A scar means I survived.'
—*Chris Cleave*

The survival rate of stage-IV ovarian cancer, according to the American Cancer Society, is only 19 per cent.[1] But I am still here—alive—despite not being expected to live. In a way, I defied my genes, my past turmoil and the dips and the valleys of my life. I do not know what worked for me, but something obviously did.

This perhaps means that anybody can be in that 19 per cent group. So please do not let go of hope. To all those who are diagnosed with cancer, fearing it or battling it, let me put your mind at rest. Cancer is *not* a death sentence. There is hope. Medical science has advanced and research is going on around the world to get to the root of cancer. Just as we have created a polio-free world, maybe we will soon have a cancer-free world. Many more people are living with the disease now than in the olden days. So please hold on to hope.

---

[1] 'Survival Rates for Ovarian Cancer, by Stage', American Cancer Society, https://www.cancer.org/cancer/ovarian-cancer/detection-diagnosis-staging/survival-rates.html.

Look at your life closely. Perhaps cancer is your wake-up call to simply change your life's lenses? To live life differently? Perhaps it is an opportunity to bring back harmony and health into your life? Could it be that your condition is not a disease, but a dis-ease? Perhaps your body is longing to be in harmony.

I urge you to use this as an opportunity to examine your lifestyle carefully and invite harmony back into your life.

Live Mindfully in the Here and Now

Stress has become rampant in each person's life today. Just look around you. Everything is in frantic motion; everyone is filled with anxiety. I see many youngsters rushing to meet deadlines. People are living like robots—performing tasks mechanically. Unfortunately, I too was living life in a rush and look where I landed.

It took cancer to make me more mindful of everything around me. To live life one day at a time. So today I make a conscious effort to be truly present in each moment. I try to be mindful all the time.

Mindfulness is a state achieved by awareness of the present moment, while watching our thoughts or 'mind chatter' which generates feelings and bodily sensations. When you become aware of your anxieties and bodily sensations you realize that you can take a different course.

Let me share some things that have worked for me positively. These practices helped me get through my dark times. Perhaps they could help you too.

Introspect, dig deep and get clarity

Introspection has truly worked for me. I simply dip within and find my answers.

Re-evaluate your life. Sit quietly, pay attention and get clarity.

On a scale of 1 to 10 where are you now? In your job, relationships, finance, health?

Remember, it is important to be honest. Please be mindful of the fact that we tend to lie to ourselves more than to others!

Be kind

Be kind to yourself. We are often too harsh with ourselves, so please be kind. If you find yourself having slipped in any area, please put yourself back on track gently. The keyword here is 'gently'.

Stay committed to change

Focus on change. Change is the most difficult thing to do as we are habitual beings and tend to follow certain patterns. Most of these patterns are unconscious. That is why, even when we want to change our unhealthy habits, it becomes difficult. But try to remain committed to change, however difficult it may seem.

Please be focused on why you wanted to change your unhealthy habits in the first place.

Develop an Attitude of Gratitude

How many of us feel deeply grateful for the blessings we receive each day in the form of basics such as food, shelter, clothing and the people who support us in our day-to-day life? Perhaps, over time, we take these for granted and somewhere, begin feeling entitled.

Cancer made me awash with gratitude. It opened before me the treasures of everyday living. I felt like a child being shown a treasure house and set free to discover it.

Cancer taught me to pay attention to the taste of the fruits I ate—the juiciness of apples and the tartness of lemons. It taught me to choose and enjoy nourishing foods. It taught me to marvel at the magnificence of sunrises and sunsets, to be awed by the star-studded night skies and to be fascinated by the shapes of clouds. It taught me to appreciate the colours of all the marvellous birds I saw flying around and rejoice at god's handiwork. It taught me to pay more attention to the expressions people wear every day, the marks of their struggles and the laugh lines imprinted by life.

In short, it taught me to appreciate minute things. I found beauty in mundaneness. Having noticed all this wealth around me, I was overcome with gratitude.

Develop Positivity, Drop Negativity

A positive attitude, they say, can create more miracles than any wonder drug. The Law of Attraction also explains that one gets more of what one focuses on. So why not create a beautiful life for oneself by focusing on the positive?

Of course, life is all about difficulties, ups and downs and disappointments. But it is also about success, happiness and fulfilled dreams once we overcome our struggles.

Negativity is injurious to health. Yet many of us keep dwelling on the negative and see only problems instead of opportunities in every situation. Is it any wonder that the lives of such people are joyless and unhappy because of this attitude?

Post cancer, I switched my attention to positivity and remained focused on staying afloat emotionally. Of course it was a struggle. A web search on the outcomes of my kind of cancer threw up a lot of depressing information. But having made up my mind to remain positive, I could focus on the life I would live *after* getting cured.

Even now, I consciously seek out positive stories about people and fight the mind's tendency to dip into the negative and the depressing. Have you tried this? When you consciously make an effort to develop such a mind state, you are rewarded with what you are looking for—positivity.

There is an age-old Native American parable that I would like to narrate to you. An old Cherokee indigenous man was teaching his grandson about life. 'A fight is going on inside me,' he said to the boy. 'It is a terrible fight and it is between two wolves. One is evil—he is anger, envy, sorrow, regret, greed, arrogance, self-pity, guilt, resentment, inferiority, lies, false pride, superiority and ego.' He continued, 'The other is good—he is joy, peace, love, hope, serenity, humility, kindness, benevolence, empathy, generosity, truth, compassion and faith. The same fight is going on inside you—and inside every other person, too.' The grandson thought about it for a minute and then asked his grandfather, 'Which wolf will win?' The old Cherokee simply replied, 'The one you feed.'

We Are Not Just Our Physical Body

I had a wonderful session with my psychotherapist after cancer. He helped me navigate and discover my childhood's unresolved issues. Once these issues are brought out from our unconscious (subconscious) into our conscious, it is our job to take the right action.

I've done enough reading to understand how the mind and body are interconnected and intertwined. One affects the other in ways we cannot even fathom. We simply cannot ignore one aspect and expect to be cured fully. Only when we treat these as one wondrous unit can we expect to live a healthy life. In fact, a lot of scientists have done experiments on the placebo effect and there are many theories to confirm this. This is why I felt it was important to work on my own issues with a psychotherapist.

The ultimate goal of holistic healing—something I strongly believe and support—is wholeness. The power of holistic healing is now being accepted and understood by medical science too. It gives me immense joy to see that this understanding is now helping shape modern-day medicine as well.

We Are Interconnected, Not Separate; We Are Powerful, Not Helpless

As a novice and amateur explorer, I began reading about life, death and the natural laws governing them. It was then that I stumbled upon the intriguing topic of quantum physics. Quantum physics is a complex subject which I will dare to offer a simplistic explanation for.

In physics, this is a fundamental theory. It deals with the study of atoms and subatomic particles which are the smallest scales of energy. The Merriam-Webster dictionary explains quantum mechanics as a branch of physics that deals with the structure and behaviour of very small pieces of matter.

Danish physicist Niels Henrik David Bohr received the Nobel Prize in Physics in 1922 for his introductory work in the area of understanding and explaining quantum theory and atomic structure. 'Anyone not shocked by quantum mechanics has not yet understood it,' he said.

This science has blown away the myth of humans being the dominant creations on earth. The truth is we share the same composition at the atomic and molecular level with everything—with the tree outside our window and the insect on the grass. We are made of the same stuff. This means that not only are we humans connected to each other, but also to everything around us. We are not superior. We are same. In fact the chair on which you are sitting right now has the same composition as your body. What a humbling discovery!

Our interconnectedness has been backed and supported by many studies, as well as by the discourses of many philosophers down the ages. This completely shatters our illusion of separateness. In his book *Moving through Parallel Worlds to Achieve Your Dreams*, Kevin Michel writes: 'You are deluded if you think that the world around you is a physical construct separate from your own mind.'

We are all deeply interconnected, regardless of our geographical distance, race or religion. Because of this, we get impacted at a deep level by any drastic event that occurs in any part of the world. Studies in quantum physics validate these beliefs. This is also one of the concepts I learnt at Oneness University. Those interested to know more might like to watch the documentary *What the Bleep!?: Down the Rabbit Hole* (2006), directed by William Arntz, Betsy Chasse and Mark Vicente.

We are all energy in motion (e-motion) and can impact life around us. It also means that we can impact our lives by the thoughts we think. My favourite author Dr Bruce Lipton has explained this theory beautifully in his books *Wisdom of Your Cells* and *The Biology of Belief*.

He has explained cell biology in a fascinating way. This new area of study takes us from the victim to the creator mode. He says that we are powerful enough to create and unfold the lives we lead. He says, 'The moment you change your perception is the moment you rewrite the chemistry of your body.'

According to him, gene activity can change on a daily basis. If the perception in our mind gets reflected in the chemistry of our body, and if our nervous system reads and interprets the environment and then controls the blood's chemistry, then we can literally change the fate of our cells by altering our thoughts. I was bewildered. I found this to be hugely empowering!

I would like to quote Dr Lipton's beautiful piece of wisdom, 'If humans were to model the lifestyle displayed by healthy community of cells, our societies and our planet would be more peaceful and vital.'

Accepting Death as a Natural Process of Life

All of us fear it, but none will escape it. We all know that everything that is born must die. Life is believed to have four stages—birth, ageing, sickness and death. Once one accepts the inevitability of death, we get closer to reality.

Yet most of us deny, refuse to talk about it or sweep it under the carpet. Death remains a hush-hush, ominous, taboo word.

Cancer made me face my own mortality. I realized that the fear of death was crippling my emotions. I told myself that this fear was unnecessary since death was a natural process of life. I understood that life was finite and limited. That calmed me down a little.

My death will come when the time is right. So why not accept it instead of spending my days fretting about it or remaining fearful of it?

Of course, on my wish list is the desire to die in a peaceful, dignified manner, whenever my time comes. For death is indeed a natural cycle of life.

Cancer also gave me the understanding that the only time we have been given on earth is the interval between birth and death. So why not live our days fully and meaningfully?

My journey towards understanding the concept of death led me to reading many books. I discovered that Hinduism views death as something spiritual. It is here that we find the concept of rebirth and reincarnation of souls. According to Hinduism, death is regarded as a natural process in the existence of soul as a separate entity. Hindus believe that when a person dies, the soul travels for some time to another world and finally returns again to continue its journey on earth. The Sanskrit word for this is *antarabhava*—the intermediate, transitional state between death and rebirth. And moksha is the ultimate goal of the soul's journey. It refers to various forms of emancipation, liberation and release in Hinduism, Buddhism, Jainism and Sikhism. Moksha refers to freedom from samsara, the cycle of death and rebirth. Buddhists also call it nirvana.

My curiosity to learn more led me to a fascinating and extremely profound book—*The Tibetan Book of Living and Dying* by Sogyal Rinpoche.

It was in this book that I came across the word bardo. According to the Oxford dictionary, bardo is a state of existence between death and rebirth, varying in length according to a person's conduct in life and manner of, or age at, death.

Bardo (antarabhava in Sanskrit) is the period after death and before one's next birth when one's consciousness is not connected with the physical body. Yet one experiences a variety of phenomena in this state. I was fascinated by this concept and am still in the process of understanding it at a deep spiritual level. When my bardo comes, I wish to be prepared for it.

I have heard a fascinating story about ancient Egyptians. They believed that upon death, the soul was asked two profound questions. Those are the ones I wish to ask you now.

The first question is, 'Did you bring joy?'
The second is, 'Did you find joy?'

I urge you to read and ponder over these questions deeply. Many times over. After you have done so, why not go about implementing them in your lives? Let us not wait for death to ask us these questions. Let's build our present lives on working on answering these questions happily.

To Sum It Up

Cancer became my teacher. It taught me to seek out help in various aspects influencing my health. It led me to learn yoga and pranayama and it encouraged me to deepen my spiritual understanding by going to Oneness University. It taught me not to shy away from seeking advice from experts. I sought advice from my life coach Santhosh Babu as well as a spiritual teacher named Kiran-ji (earlier called Naman-ji). I have also become more mindful of the company I keep. I initiate positivity and ensure that my work environment remains healthy. My doctors remain my go-to people whenever I need to take a new step towards my health. For they are the magicians who saved me. And that makes me feel deeply grateful towards them.

Most importantly, cancer made me focus on my behaviour as a person. I have worked hard and continue to work mindfully at becoming the best version of myself—emotionally, spiritually and physically. I grew to become the kind of person I would like to be with. Liking your own company is the first step towards healing.

So I have a question for you. Are you the kind of person you would like to be with? Are you the friend people would seek out for company?

I hope the answer is yes.

All the best!

20

Not Only through the Male Gaze

'Just as the pure white lotus flower blooms unsoiled in muddy water, our lives, which are supremely noble, can continue to shine even amid life's harshest realities.'

—*Daisaku Ikeda*

The other day, a man wrote on my Twitter handle: 'You look old!' It sounded as if being old was a curse.

I felt like writing back, 'Of course I am old. I will soon turn fifty. So what?'

This year, in 2018, I rang in my forty-eighth birthday in style by inviting several of my close friends from the film industry. I had the five-star venue decked up enchantingly with flowers and made it a joyous white-themed party. So much for a birthday at this age? Of course! I have stared at death from such close range that each year added to my life is a cause for celebration.

And this brings me to the issue of women and ageing, a subject I feel strongly about.

One of the infallible laws of nature is that every human will pass through four stages—birth, ageing, sickness and death. Some will experience the ravages of time in a harsher way, while for others it may not be so. But they will experience it.

Despite knowing this, as a society, we judge women using a stricter yardstick. We expect them to be walking around like ornamental, fragrant flowers, looking fresh, breathtaking and desirable throughout their lives. This is particularly true about our expectations from celebrities.

Why don't we judge men as harshly? An older man is 'seasoned and mature', whereas a woman is 'old and past her prime'.

What this does is put too much of pressure on women to remain youthful for as long as they can, often forcing them to go to great lengths to achieve these elusive standards. As for men, have you seen how silly an aged man looks with a young beauty on his arms? And have you noticed the sense of pride he feels in having it all—money, status, young women—despite his paunch and bald head?

It is as if ageing men are trapped in a room, surrounded by mirrors on all sides, each reflecting the age they imagine themselves to have frozen at. I do not mean to be critical of anyone. Each one to his own. If that makes you happy, go ahead. But why have different standards for women?

This attitude seeps into our films too, where a man in his fifties can romance a girl in her twenties, but a heroine quickly loses her 'shelf life'. As if we were a carton of perishables! This is why very few meaningful roles are being written for women past their prime.

But things are changing, though slowly. There is reason for hope. I picked up the role of a middle-aged woman in *Dear Maya* (2017) in which the whole film revolved around her character. Before that, I played a middle-aged woman in a Kannada film. This year too, in 2018, I did two movies. Though they were short roles, they were powerful ones. Next year, I am acting in two movies and they both have excellent scripts with strong women characters. Of course such scripts are few and far between, but that suits me fine.

In between, I get time to do the things I love and realize my other dreams and aspirations. Some of these are: going to Kathmandu and staying with my family; working on my book; trekking and hiking; doing cancer awareness programmes, cleaning River Bagmati and so on. Professionally, I am largely content. However, I still long to see a woman past her forties playing the protagonist. I want to see that happening in my lifetime.

I would love to see forty-plus women blossoming to their full potential—career-wise, family-wise and in every aspect of their lives. And yes, I would love to have more roles with excellent scripts and great directors.

I believe that just as a fruit ripens in season, age brings with it more beauty. A woman gets blessed with deeper perspectives, maturer outlooks and more layers to her personality that were earlier unexplored and unexpressed. Having lived through life's twisted turns, she becomes nothing short of a marvel of nature worked on by Time. I mention here six inspirational women from three countries who have shaped me—Nepal's Sushila Ama (my grandmother) and my mother; India's Sarojini Naidu and Maharani Gayatri Devi; and Maya Angelou as well as Oprah Winfrey of the US.

I believe in the concept of celebrating life's every season. It takes sunshine and showers to make us blossom fully. And when we have blossomed, the skin *does* begin to sag a little, the wrinkles *do* appear around the mouth and eyes. I say, it is okay! That's how it's meant to be!

As women, let us wear these 'wisdom lines' as our badges of pride and honour, of marks left behind after fighting life's battles bravely. And let us see the streaks of lightning in our hair as symbols of victory and triumph. Aren't soldiers proud of theirs wounds and scars? So why should we get shamed into hiding ours?

Cancer has flooded me with new wisdom, new realizations and new questions.

My resolve now is to live a life of moderation and balance. When this book hits the stands, you might just see me everywhere, urging you to live such a life too in the interest of your own health. I reiterate: Health is our most precious possession.

And now, I have a few pointers dedicated to my women readers. Like a flooded river leaves behind rich deposits of silt, cancer left behind many learnings for me. It brought calmness and mindfulness. It taught me to never devalue myself. To be grateful for each precious moment and live it fully.

Please take what I write below as precious lessons I have picked up from my life's journey. The insights may not be new. You may know them already, but we women do need to be reminded of their importance once in a while.

Stop the Blame Game

It seems blaming ourselves is inbuilt into our systems. As if guilt trips were not bad enough, we happily take on ourselves the blame of everything going wrong in our lives. Call it years of conditioning. Evolved as I dare consider myself to be, even I have to consciously watch myself from overthinking if I brought cancer upon myself.

I? Causing it? There, you see?

I remember Dr Makker telling me: 'If at all your cancer recurs, do not blame yourself as you did not cause it.' I am certain one of her women patients (or several) may have shared with her the blame game they whipped themselves with.

So ladies, I urge you to drop this toxin right now!

Banish Negativity

Experience has taught me that there is a strong connection between the body, mind and spirit. Dr Narula is my rakhi brother. Both he and his wife, Zeena-ji, were a strong support system during my treatment. Dr Narula's advice and my own research have taught me that non-communicable diseases are lifestyle illnesses.

A healthy lifestyle can keep many diseases away. I build my motivational talks around the country based on this wisdom. An acidic body becomes host to illnesses. Dwelling constantly on negativity directly impacts health.

Emotion, or e-motion, is energy in motion. Allow it to come, but also allow it to drift away. Emotions like anger, jealousy and anxiety, if harboured too long in the body, make it acidic. And that's where the problem starts. Do not try being a people-pleaser at the cost of your health. It's just not worth it. Stay in balance and always remain aware of maintaining harmony between the mind, body and spirit.

So ladies, surround yourself with positive friends and influences. Flood your life with sunshine!

Taking Responsibility of Your Health Parameters

I now realize how unaware I was of the negative effect IVF injections could have on someone who was BRCA-1 positive. Dr Chi had told me that this cancer affects older women and he was surprised I had been struck by it in my forties itself. How I wish I had informed myself better!

So ladies, read up and arm yourself with knowledge. Your body is the only vehicle you have to travel through in this life!

Look up to Yourself

When I was at my lowest phase in life, a horrible picture of mine hit the newspapers. I was coming out of a pub drunk and the camera flashlights had caught me. I looked like a stricken deer caught in the headlights of a car.

I hated the way I looked. Fat and messed up. But this was not the only time. YouTube videos had shamed me earlier.

I decided this had to stop. I called out to the little girl inside me who had surprised everyone with top grades when taunted. I nudged awoke the little girl who, even in moments of distress, had refused to make a public spectacle of herself. She would shed tears behind the closed doors of the bathroom. I saw this young actress who had emerged strong in the face of adversity several times. I marvelled at the woman who had survived cancer so commendably. I felt a rush of pride for her. And suddenly I loved this girl-woman.

Ladies, please cast a fond look back at your journey and pat yourself on the back right now!

Nurture Yourself

Don't sacrifice yourself at the family altar. Don't spread yourself until it hurts. You are the fulcrum around which your family revolves. You need to be in good health for you to take care of your family.

Cancer has taught me to not seek validation from another person. If you do, you will get disappointed often. Life has now taught me to use my inner compass and judgement to decide my steps forward. I will do nothing to dishonour myself.

So ladies, make self-love and self-nurturing your mantras!

Heal Yourself and Keep Growing

Books, art therapy and music have become the pillars of my life. Art therapy uses therapeutic techniques as a creative method of expression. For me, it is all about expressing myself. I feel any emotion, pain or anxiety, if unexpressed, becomes toxic.

The music I listen to is always soothing, meditative and calming. Instrumental music, particularly the flute and the piano, are my favourites. I love listening to nature's sounds too—of the sea, of the wind, of the rainforest. I am also a fan of jazz music. When in New York, I love going to jazz clubs. I love the way the music resembles a story and has a beginning, middle and end. I enjoy the way one piece flows into another and becomes an enchanting story, staying on in your memory for a long time.

At the end of this book, you will find a list of some of the resources that have helped me grow. I have derived a lot of strength and wisdom from them. I can happily say that I am strong, calm and peaceful because of these resources.

I mention below some insights I have gleaned from my self-search. I could tide over my dark times because of these precious gems of wisdom. Perhaps they might help you too.

Keep checking these four quotients regularly:

- Growth Quotient: Are you holding fossilized ideas and attitudes? Are you growing each day in mind and spirit?

- Fulfilment Quotient: You are taking care of all those you are expected to nurture. You are being responsible as best as you can. Do you feel resentful or fulfilled doing so?
- Authenticity Quotient: Are you suppressing the real you to fulfil others' expectations and dreams? What about yours?
- Freedom Quotient: Do you feel free in mind, body and spirit? Are you free to reimagine, reinvent and realign yourself whenever you wish?

When you answer these honestly, you realize that over time you have become a true woman. And that discovery will be the biggest gift to yourself.

Ladies, let us rejoice in the ripeness of age and glow in the radiance of acceptance. Life is meant to be a celebration. Let's begin celebrating ourselves—wrinkles and all. Let us stop chasing perfection.

We form one half of humanity. We have given birth to those very men who often run us down, ravage us and feel 'entitled' to dominate over us. Worse, we endanger our own species right from the womb, because we feel we are not good enough to be accepted in this male-dominated world.

Can we change our attitude to ourselves? Can we first become fiercely proud of who we are? Can we begin supporting our fellow sisters as our own, instead of running them down? Can we build, not tear down? Can you imagine what a world it would be in which women become strong supporters of each other? There's so much power in that!

But for that to happen, we need to first accept our worth. To recognize that we are limitless, borderless, infinite and simply unstoppable. Can we become the change we expect society to reflect?

Let us not expect others to define us. We are the seekers and the sought; we are the givers and the gifts; we are the creation and the creators.

In short, we are *woman*.

This is not a word, phrase or sentence. It is the kind, compassionate, nurturing, healing power of the universe.

It is complete.

Living the New Me

'Whenever you find yourself doubting how far you can go, just remember how far you have come. Remember everything you have faced, all the battles you have won, and all the fears you have overcome.'

—*Unknown*

Months of intense inner gardening has revealed a new friend to me—*Manisha*. With this joyous, wiser, confident, glorious new being by my side, I am ready to take on the world. Ready for the challenges life will unfold before me. I have now developed a new skill set to handle it.

This new me has given birth to the 'Koirala woman' inside me. That grit remained with me while acting. I remember my screen test for 1942: *A Love Story*. Veteran film-maker Vidhu Vinod Chopra had called me to do a scene. But to my disappointment, at the end of it he remarked: 'Manisha, you were shit. You're a terrible actress.'

This was not acceptable to me. The warrior woman inside me had been challenged. I requested him to give me twenty-four hours to come back for a second chance. Back home, I practised my lines passionately, over and over again, until my mother became distressed at my state.

'What are you doing to yourself? It's okay if you don't get this movie. Don't kill yourself over it.'

Next day, I poured my soul into my performance. Vidhu remained silent for long, as if in a daze. And then he said the words that were music to my ears: 'If this is the heart and soul that you promise to put into each scene of my movie, I will sign you up instead of Madhuri Dixit. Manisha, yesterday, you were at zero. You are at a hundred today.'

And that is how I got signed for 1942—a movie that became a box-office hit and had critics describing me as a powerhouse of talent.

Reinvented, renewed and realigned, I have now set clear boundaries around me. My constant struggle is to shatter my hardness and yet not become vulnerable.

Do I still want a boyfriend? Of course I do!

But now I will allow someone into my sacred space only after putting him through a thorough check. I refuse to experience another heartbreak. So what is it I'm looking for?

Someone who is my equal, understands me, respects everything I have been through. A partner who has resolved or is in the process of resolving his own issues. Someone who is willing to help me work through mine and is open to letting me help him through his. In short, a mature, spiritual, financially stable, accomplished good-looking man. In that order. Too much to ask for? Maybe. Will I find him? I don't know. Will I compromise on this? Never.

Until then, I will remain self-contained, whole and happy in my own company, much like a precious oyster in its pretty shell.

So has cancer changed me? Yes.

In the morning of my newness, I find myself washed of unnecessary trappings—just like rain washes out yesterday's grime. Designer clothes and bags are mere possessions now, not obsessions. Relationships are precious, not merely timepass. Drama is something I restrict only to my screen performances. I went through immense pain to cleanse my emotional life of negativity and toxic people, situations and relationships. In place of this clutter, my day is now filled with health and nutrition regimens, exercise, yoga and pranayama. I have restarted my career in films. I am deeply grateful for this chance, just as I am deeply grateful for anything life gives me now.

If I was a weak tree earlier, ready to topple at the first strong breeze that blew at me, I am now a deep-rooted banyan. I have branched out in many directions, expressing all my multifaceted sides.

As a motivational speaker, I share precious life lessons at various schools, hospitals and organizations.

As a United Nations Population Fund (UNFPA) goodwill ambassador, I have seen the enormous suffering people lived through and are living through after the Nepal earthquake in 2015. I have done my bit to coordinate and provide relief work in the affected areas. A lot, however, still remains to be done.

As a social worker, I am also actively involved in working with organizations to promote women's rights and the prevention of violence against women and human trafficking of Nepali girls for prostitution.

I feel expanded in heart, generous in spirit. It is my time under the sun now. I am burning with the desire to give back to society.

I think cancer came into my life as a gift. My vision is sharper, my mind clearer, my perspective realigned. I have succeeded in transforming my passive-aggressive anger and anxiety into more peaceful expressions. But hey, I am still human! So they do leak out sometimes. This means I am still a work in progress. But I am definitely a better person now—kinder, more generous and disarmingly genuine.

I have changed from the inside. And so has my world.

I remember being frightened at my re-entry into films.

Would the audience accept me? Would they write me off?

That's when I read the empowering words of Daisaku Ikeda, 'Life is filled with potential that is truly unfathomable . . . That is why we must never write anyone off. In particular, we mustn't put boundaries on our own potential. In most cases, our so-called limitations are nothing more than our own decision to limit ourselves.'

At first it was difficult for me to take on the role of a character artist as I had been used to playing the heroine. Then I saw the blessing in this. Having plunged into the depths of my emotions, I could now express the intricate complexities, deeper nuances and profounder layers of each character.

I began my second innings hesitatingly, with a Kannada film. And then, in 2017, I was offered *Dear Maya*—a dark film about an elderly woman whose face mirrors her intense feelings. Drawing from the depths of my own darkness, I performed like never before. Would I have been able to enact such a role before I had been diagnosed with cancer? Maybe yes! Who knows?

I no longer sign films mindlessly. I do so only if they are meaningful and intense.

In December 2016, casting director Mukesh Chhabria called me up in Kathmandu. He informed me that Raju sir (Hirani) wanted me to play the role of the iconic Nargis, who had tragically lost her life to pancreatic cancer at the age of fifty-one.

No! My heart screamed.

Everything about this offer seems frightening. How can I play a cancer patient? How can I handle those fears again? How can I depict the talented

Nargis-ji? How can I play the mother of Ranbir Kapoor? Isn't he just a decade younger to me?

Still undecided, I flew to Mumbai ten days later and decided to visit Raju sir's film set.

My meeting warmed my heart. I was welcomed back with immense love and joy. What a positive environment greeted me! The film set overflowed with happiness and team spirit.

No wonder Raju Hirani's films capture goodness and warm-heartedness so beautifully on screen. These feelings are born out of the atmosphere he cultivates while shooting.

Instinctively, I went up to Raju sir and smiled my acceptance.

Working with Raju sir, mingling with Imtiaz, talking to the supremely talented and sweet Ranbir, I realized how cinema has changed from our times. It is now so open, warm, friendly and safe. What is paramount is a good script, a talented crew and a great product.

Within this foundation, an original, unique work is born. This is the reason so much experimentation and diversity can be seen in films today.

In short, I love this new 'film home' that has sprouted out here and do want to continue being a part of it. I hope I have just showcased the tip of the iceberg of my talent. The real stuff still remains unexplored within me.

My needs are different now. The new me will not settle for mere existence. I will reach out for adventures that warm the soul. I will reach out for what makes my cells dance with joy. I need to keep growing. I have finally embraced life and I think it has embraced me back.

Epilogue

It's been six years now since I have been cancer-free.

As I near the end of my fourth decade on this planet, I rejoice at this second chance at life. I feel my life is beginning only now.

The loaded word intezaar, which earlier spelt doom and foreboding for me during those endless hours I spent waiting for my reports and the doctors' verdicts, has now transformed into a positive, hopeful word.

With bated breath, I await the miracles, the possibilities and the magic tomorrow promises.

Acknowledgements

I have always believed that I am a spiritual being going through a human experience. Therefore, each person who has come into my life has been a lesson, each encounter a blessing.

But since we are all handiworks of those we feel close to and feel appreciative of, I would like to mention a few people who have made my life beautiful. Do forgive me if I have inadvertently left out some names.

Before I thank anyone, I would like to thank my beloved parents who were with me through thick and thin, standing strong, like the Rock of Gibraltar.

Immense gratitude also to my brother, Siddharth (I can never repay Bhai for his love and care in this lifetime), Yulia and my niece, Yamini.

My heartfelt thanks to Dr Dennis Chi, Dr Vicky Makker, Dr Madhu Ghimire, Dr Suresh Advani and Dr Prakash Khoobchandani.

Sri Bhagavan and the Oneness team for sending me healing *deeksha* and giving me the tools to handle life.

Pilot Baba and all his disciples.

Sahara Shree for his kindness.

Chetna Di and Praveen Da for being my support in a new country.

Dr Meena, Dr Suresh Jhanawar and Sabrina Jhanawar for being supportive in a myriad ways.

Dr Mukul Singh, Dr Dipika Bajaj, Dr Meera Chatterjee and Kumy Khanna Bhasin.

Dr Narayan Naidu will always remain larger than life for me. He spent long hours sitting by my bedside, infusing me with hope, strength and grit, despite his crazy busy schedule. His inspirational words gave me the courage to face my ordeal.

Dr Jagat Narula and Dr Navneet Narula for consistently being my support.

Shiva (for getting me fresh water fish in New York!) and Biru for always being there for me.

Anu, my cousin Mona, Mridula Aunty, Lulu Rana, Adrish Chakravarty, Sudhir Vaishnav, Yasir and Vicky, Supriya, Himanshu–Mandira and their joyous kids.

My late Shail Mama.

Rachna Chhachi and Simi Singh Juneja for helping me write this book in its initial stages. Rachna has her own naturopathy centre and heals her patients with a lot of passion. Simi, blessed with the ability to express well, helped me dig deep into my core and become brave enough to confront some of my memories. She made me feel safe during my darkest phase. Without the help of these two ladies, this book would have been incomplete.

Gratitude to the one who broke my heart but taught me precious life lessons.

Deep appreciation to those friends who were there with me in New York in spirit—Avinash Adik, Amit Ashar, Srinivas Bhanshyam, Gulshan Grover and Shatrughan Sinha-ji.

I want to thank Eric Mistry, my psychotherapist, as well as Santhosh Babu for helping me overcome my fear of public speaking and encouraging me to share my story.

A big thank you to my countless fans and well-wishers. You are, therefore I am.

Thank you to Neelam Kumar for helping me finish this book. Actually, this was her idea. Thank you, Neelam, for putting words to my feelings. This book would not have happened without your brilliance.

How can I not thank Gurveen Chadha of Penguin Random House for showing immense patience through the creation of each draft of my book?

Finally, a big thank you to life itself.

Manisha Koirala

This book has been a work of intense love and deep pain.

Let me explain.

I was handed over a horror script as my life—widowhood at thirty-five, single parenting, limited resources, challenges of daily living and then breast cancer. Not once but twice.

My life has been a struggle to prove my middle-school teacher's prediction wrong that I would never be able to learn the English language. I went on to write eight successful books.

I met Manisha in 2015. She very generously wrote a foreword to my book on cancer. Back then, we had planned to write her book, but it finally got written in 2018.

During the writing of this book, I realized what a perfectionist Manisha is. She would go through every sentence, every emotion and every phrase and discuss whether it should or should not be in her book.

I waited for her characteristic 'Babe, thumbs-up' at the end of each chapter as we read it through. I had earlier been dazzled by her screen presence. But what I saw close-up was even more dazzling. She is brave, vulnerable, honest and very real. These are the qualities that get reflected in this book.

Writing Manisha's journey, particularly the chemotherapy emotions, compelled me to confront and deal with mine.

Towards the end of writing this book, both of us went for our check-ups and received an 'asymptomatic', all-clear report!

That's how much effort and heart have gone into creating this book. I hope you find it rich in intimacy, imagery, customs, traditions, cancer insights, spirituality and gentle humour.

I strongly feel that our society needs to change the narrative on survivors. There seems to be no space for us. Yet many more of us are now living rich lives—joyously, optimistically and resiliently.

It is my earnest prayer that Manisha's book becomes an inspiring example of this and leads the way.

Thank you, Manisha and Gurveen Chadha, for giving me this opportunity.

Neelam Kumar

Books and Resources: My Portable Magic

Here's a list of some of my favourite readings, audios and videos. I like to think of them as my portable magic.

Books

Srimad Bhagavad Gita. Commentary by Swami B.G. Narasingha. Bangalore: Gosai Publishers, 2011.

Hay, Louise L. *You Can Heal Your Life*. London: Hay House, 1984.

Hay, Louise L. *The Power Is Within You*. London: Hay House, 1991.

Dyer, Dr Wayne W., *Change Your Thoughts, Change Your Life: Living the Wisdom of The Tao*. California: Hay House, 2008.

Dyer, Dr Wayne W. *Being in Balance: 9 Principles for Creating Habits to Match Your Desires*. California: Hay House, 2016.

Tuchowska, Marta. *Committed to Wellness, Fitness and a Healthy Lifestyle: How to Unleash Your Inner Motivation, Change Your Mind and Transform Your Body Fast*. California: CreateSpace Independent Publishing Platform, 2015.

Lipton, Bruce H. *The Biology of Belief*. California: Hay House, 2016

Dyer, Dr Wayne W. *Wishes Fulfilled: Mastering the Art of Manifesting*. California: Hay House, 2013.

Chronister, Kim. *Fit Mentality: The Ultimate Guide to Stop Binge Eating: Achieve the Mindset for the Fit Body You Want.* California: CreateSpace Independent Publishing Platform, 2015.

Boehmer, Tami. *Miracle Survivors: Beating the Odds of Incurable Cancer.* New York: Skyhorse Publishing, 2014.

Siegel, Bernie and Jennifer Sander. *Faith, Hope and Healing: Inspiring Lessons Learned from People Living with Cancer.* New Jersey: Wiley, 2009.

Connealy, Leigh Erin. *The Cancer Revolution: A Ground Breaking Program to Reverse and Prevent Cancer.* Boston, MA: Da Capo Lifelong Books, 2017.

Moorjani, Anita. *Dying to Be Me: My Journey from Cancer, to Near Death, to True Healing.* California: Hay House, 2012.

Armstrong, Lance and Sally Jenkins. *It's Not about the Bike: My Journey Back to Life.* New York: Putnam, 2000.

James, John W. and Russell Friedman. *The Grief Recovery Handbook.* San Francisco: HarperCollins, 2009.

Byron, Katie. *The Work of Byron Katie.* Ebook. 2014. http://thework.com/sites/thework/downloads/little_book/English_LB.pdf.

Audio Books

Goodman, Anthony A. *Lifelong Health: Achieving Optimum Well-Being at Any Age.* The Great Courses, 2010. Audio CD; 18 hrs and 15 mins.

Hawkins, Dr David. *Healing: Achieve Total Wellness through Higher Levels of Consciousness.* Nightingale-Conant Corporation, 2010. Audio CD.

Lipton, Bruce H. *The Wisdom of Your Cells: How Your Beliefs Control Your Biology*. Sounds True, 2006. Audio CD.

Blogs

Carr, Kris. *Kris Carr* (blog). https://kriscarr.com.

Ray, Lisa. *Yellow Diaries* (blog). http://blog.lisaray.com.

Zane, Shafin De. *Redefine Your Reality* (blog). www.redefineyourreality.com.

Your own journal, waiting to be written by you